(eSRI)

The Economic and Social Research Institute

The Economic and Social Research Institute (ESRI) is a non-profit organisation which was founded in 1960 as the Economic Research Institute. The Institute is a private company, limited by guarantee, and enjoys full academic independence. It is governed by a Council consisting of 32 members who are representative of business, trade unions, government departments, state agencies, universities and other research institutes.

D1279851

The National Maternity Hospital

The National Maternity Hospital was founded in 1894 primarily to serve the poor of the surrounding districts. Since its foundation it has grown to become one of the busiest maternity hospitals in Europe, and the busiest in Ireland. The Hospital is a voluntary institution incorporated by a Royal Charter in 1903. In addition to its maternity services, it has a large gynaecological unit, and has the largest unit in the country for the care of women with gynaecological cancer. Students from University College Dublin and the Royal College of Surgeons in Ireland attend the Hospital for undergraduate education. The Survey on Women's Health Needs formed part of the Hospital's centenary activities in 1994.

Women and Health Care in Ireland

Knowledge, Attitudes and Behaviour

Miriam M. Wiley
Barry Merriman

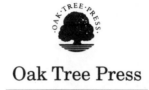

Oak Tree Press

Dublin

in association with

The Economic and Social Research Institute

Oak Tree Press
Merrion Building
Lower Merrion Street
Dublin 2, Ireland

A catalogue record of this book is
available from the British Library.

ISBN 1-86076-025-2

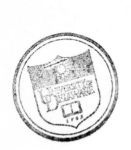

Contents

Contents vii

List of Tables

The Authors

MIRIAM M. WILEY, PhD, is Senior Research Officer and Head of the Health Policy Research Centre at the Economic and Social Research Institute.

BARRY MERRIMAN, MA, is a researcher at the Economic and Social Research Institute.

Acknowledgements

This study is based on a national survey of women's health needs commissioned from the Economic and Social Research Institute by the National Maternity Hospital, Dublin as one contribution to the celebration of the hospital's centenary in 1994. The funding provided for the study by the Health Promotion Unit of the Department of Health and Cow & Gate Ireland Ltd. is gratefully acknowledged.

In presenting this study, we would like to express our thanks for the assistance provided by Dr Peter Boylan, Master, Ms Maeve Dwyer, Matron, Ms Peggy McGuire and colleagues on the National Maternity Hospital Advisory Committee, including Ms Anna-May Harkin from the Department of Health. Dr Ruth Barrington and her colleagues at the Department of Health involved in the development of a national policy for women's health have also been very supportive of this study. In addition, we would like to thank specifically our ESRI colleagues, Professor Kieran A. Kennedy, Dr Dorothy Watson and Dr Tony Fahey for valuable comments received on an earlier draft of the study. The assistance provided by the Survey Unit and the General Office staff at the ESRI, Ms Rachel Iredale, UCD, and Ms Noreen Kearns, UCG, is sincerely appreciated. Mr David Givens and Ms Emer Ryan, Oak Tree Press, have greatly facilitated all stages of the editing and production process. Finally, and most importantly, we would like to thank all those women throughout Ireland who took the time to participate in the national survey of women's health needs and made this study possible.

1

Introduction

What do women in the Ireland of the 1990s know about their own health needs and how do they address these needs? In the absence of a national data source on the knowledge, attitudes and behaviour of Irish women towards their health-care needs, these and other related questions could not be given meaningful consideration. This type of information base is also required if policy and service developments in areas most relevant to women's health are to be adequately informed and responsive to the priorities identified by women as being essential to the achievement and maintenance of optimal health status.

In recognising the importance of such a data source for planning for more informed policy responses to women's health-care needs, the National Maternity Hospital, Holles Street, Dublin, chose to commission a national survey of women's health needs as part of the hospital's centenary celebrations in 1994. The Economic and Social Research Institute (ESRI) was commissioned to undertake this survey, the main results of which are presented in this book.

The national survey of women's health needs commissioned by the National Maternity Hospital is the first such survey undertaken in Ireland and is also unique in the international context. As the opportunity to undertake such a survey is quite a rare occurrence, it was decided to develop the most comprehensive data base possible, given the resources available. It was also considered essential that this data base would be nationally representative so that the views of women throughout the Republic of Ireland would be adequately represented. While the development of a comprehensive and nationally representative data base on women's health needs was actively pursued, certain gaps and constraints must inevitably be recognised. One important constraint which must immediately be acknowledged is that any assessment of women's health status was outside the scope of this survey. In addition, the survey was limited to women aged between 18 and 60 years of age. While it is readily recognised that the 50 per cent of the population of Irish women who are aged under 18 and over 60 have essential needs which are specific to these age groups, the objective of comprehensiveness of coverage necessitated that the survey be limited to those aged between 18 and 60. In addition, many of the areas covered — for example antenatal and postnatal experience and attitudes to breast-feeding — would be expected to have most relevance to women in this age range. It should also be recognised, however, that many of the issues of importance to women within these age limits would also apply to women of all ages.

What this survey does provide is a unique source of information on the knowledge that Irish women possess regarding a wide range of factors essential to the achievement and maintenance of good health. This information also enables an assessment of behaviour relative to knowledge, as positive results can only be achieved if knowledge gained about health-enhancing behaviour is acted upon. Finally, prevailing attitudes to previous encounters with specific areas of health service provision and current service availability are explored with a view to determining the priorities considered important by women for the future development of particular areas of the Irish health service system. Before proceeding to a discussion of the main results presented in the chapters that follow, the conduct of the survey and the data-collection process will first be described.

Survey and Sample Selection

The survey of women's health needs was based on a national sample of women aged between 18 and 60 years. The sample was drawn from the Register of Electors from which names and addresses were drawn. A minimum age of 18 years is required for inclusion in the Register of Electors. The sample was selected on the basis of the RANSAM system, which enables the implementation of a multi-stage random sample incorporating both stratification and clustering, giving each individual on the Register an equal probability of being selected (Whelan, 1979; Keogh and Whelan, 1986). Because of the nature of the Register of Electors it was not possible to draw a female-only sample — therefore, the initial selection also included males. Any names known to be male were then removed. Where there were any ambiguous or uncertain names, it was left to the interviewers to determine the sex of the person.

The interviews were carried out between April and October 1993. Interviews were not undertaken where the individual in the target sample was male or over 60 years of age. In addition, interviews could not be conducted in certain circumstances — for example when the individual had died or moved or where addresses were found to be vacant. From an initial listing of 3,940 individuals, responses were successfully obtained from 2,988 women, or 75.8 per cent. Just 7.9 per cent of the initial sample refused to be interviewed, while 11.3 per cent were not available throughout the fieldwork, 1.8 per cent were ill and 3.2 per cent could not participate for other reasons. A response rate of 76 per cent combined with a low refusal rate of 8 per cent is indicative of a high degree of acceptance of this survey among the women contacted.

The survey questionnaire was developed by an inter-disciplinary committee established by the National Maternity Hospital to ensure that issues relevant to women's health which could realistically be addressed were included in the survey. The finalised questionnaire comprised 139 questions in 11 sections and is attached for information in Appendix 1. The areas covered by this questionnaire included nutrition, sex education, sexually transmitted diseases, family planning, maternity leave, hospital services for mothers, breast-feeding, parenting skills, gynaecology, family size and lifestyles. The questionnaire was pilot tested on a sample of 50 women in March 1993. This exercise proved to be successful with regard to the willingness of the women to participate and the feasibility of completing the questionnaire as developed. One of the interesting findings from the pilot survey was that the women interviewed requested a listing of the correct information where questions had a "right/wrong" answer. This information sheet was developed for the full-scale survey and provided to participants. A copy of this information sheet is attached in Appendix 2 for reference.

The Data

While the sample was selected to be representative of the national population, sex or age could not be controlled for when using the Register of Electors as the sampling frame. As sex and age were both classification factors for inclusion in the survey, the demographic information in the sample data had to be compared with that prevailing for the population when the survey was completed. The variables used as the basis for this assessment included the following: age, marital status, employment status, medical-card status and membership of the Voluntary Health Insurance (VHI) Board. Medical-card status for the sample was compared with the population estimates available from the General Medical Services (Payments) Board, 1992. This analysis showed that the sample was representative for this variable. VHI membership for the sample was compared with estimates of VHI membership for women, provided by the board, and was found to be representative.

The sample distributions for age and marital status were compared with information on the population of 18–60-year-old women from the 1991 Census of Population. Mainly because of under-representation in the sample of 18–19-year-olds and 60-year-olds, the sample was not considered to be fully representative of the population for this variable. When the sample distribution for marital status was compared with the population breakdown from the 1991 Census of Population, the sample was found to under-represent single women significantly and to over-represent married women. The distribution of the sample data by employment status was compared with the population estimates from the 1991 Labour Force Survey. This analysis found that the sample was comparatively over-represented with people working part-time or as relatives assisting, and under-represented with students. Given the results of the analysis conducted for these three variables, the sample was reweighted by age, marital status and employment status to ensure that valid population estimates could be derived from the data base as a whole for the population of 18–60-year-old women living in Ireland. This reweighting procedure was applied to 2,978 cases as 10 cases which were missing data on marital status and/or employment status had to be excluded from the analysis. For a small number of women in the sample, data were not available for one of the three variables which included education level, medical-card status and social class. Out of the total sample, it was not possible to assign a social class for 263 cases, 107 cases were missing data on medical-card status and 43 cases were missing data on education level. The sample size for the analysis on these variables was therefore reduced accordingly.

Following the reweighting of the sample, the distribution of women for the demographic and socioeconomic variables used in the analysis are presented in Tables 1.1 to 1.8. These tables present an interesting overview of the current demographic profile of women in the Ireland of the 1990s. While 62 per cent of women are married, almost half are engaged in home duties, with just 34 per cent working on a full-time basis. The 30 per cent of women with medical cards contrasts with the 41 per cent who have VHI membership. Only 8 per cent of women have a university qualification, while an additional 5 per cent have a qualification from an RTC or equivalent institution. The Eastern Health Board accounts for one-third of all women, while less than 40 per cent are reported to be living in a rural area. At 28 per cent, the highest proportion of women are found in the other non-manual social class while just 8 per cent are included within the higher professional group.

Table 1.1: Distribution of Women by Age Category

Age Category	Percentage
18–24	18.9
25–29	13.5
30–34	13.2
35–39	13.3
40–44	11.9
45–49	10.6
50–54	8.3
55–60	10.4

Table 1.2: Distribution of Women by Marital Status

Marital Status	Percentage
Married	62.4
Single	31.6
Married but Living Apart (not legally separated or divorced)	2.1
Divorced/Legally Separated	0.9
Widowed	2.9

Table 1.3: Distribution of Women by Employment Status

Employment Status	Percentage
Full Time*	33.7
Part Time	5.9
Unemployed	4.6
Engaged in Home Duties	47.7
Other**	8.0

*   Includes at work as relative assisting.
**   Includes student/retired/ill/disable and others not in labour force.

Table 1.4: Distribution of Women by Medical-Card Status

Medical-Card Status	Percentage
Covered by a Medical Card	30.0
Not Covered by a Medical Card	70.0

Table 1.5: Distribution of Women by VHI Membership

VHI Membership	Percentage
Member of VHI	40.7
Not a Member of VHI	59.3

Table 1.6: Distribution of Women by Education Level

Education Level	Percentage
Primary Cert/Lower	22.0
Inter/Group/Junior Cert	26.1
Leaving Cert/Matric	38.6
Qualification from RTC etc.	5.4
University Qualification	8.1

Table 1.7: Distribution of Women by Health-Board Area and Geographical Location

Health-Board Area	Percentage
East	36.6
Midland	6.0
Mid-West	8.1
North-East	9.1
North-West	7.0
South	15.9
South-East	7.6
West	9.7
Geographical Location	
Rural	39.3
Urban	60.7

Table 1.8: Distribution of Women by Social Class

Social Class	Percentage
Higher Professional, Higher Managerial; Proprietors and Farmers Farming 200 or More Acres	7.8
Lower Professional, Lower Managerial; Proprietors and Farmers Farming 100–199 Acres	20.0
Other Non-Manual and Farmers Farming 50–99 Acres	27.5
Skilled Manual and Farmers Farming 30–49 Acres	12.4
Semi-Skilled Manual and Farmers Farming Less that 30 Acres	17.1
Unskilled Manual	6.7
Unknown	8.5

The survey results presented in this publication are based on the reweighted data to ensure representativeness of the population of 18–60-year-old women in Ireland. Given the very broad scope of this survey, all of the areas investigated could not be included in a single book, though it would be hoped that subsequent publications will address those issues not considered here. In this presentation, therefore, attention has been focused on those issues which are very directly related to the personal health of women and their interaction with the health services. The chapters that follow are thus concerned with substance use and abuse among women; the receipt, source, availability and adequacy of sex education and family planning; knowledge and availability of gynaecology services and hospital services for mothers; and attitudes and approaches to breast-feeding. The conclusions and policy recommendations indicated by the information and opinions forthcoming from this study of women and health care in Ireland are summarised in the final chapter.

2

Substance Use and Abuse

Introduction

Smoking and the misuse of alcohol are major causes of morbidity for the general population. The morbidity and risk of mortality associated with these risk factors are greatly increased when women continue to smoke and abuse alcohol when pregnant, as the health of the baby is also put at risk. The Department of Health's *Health Promotion Strategy* (1995c) states that over 6,000 deaths annually in Ireland can be directly attributed to smoking. Smoking is a major risk factor for heart disease, bronchitis and emphysema, cerebrovascular disease, gastric ulcers and cancers of the mouth, throat, oesophagus, bladder and kidneys. In 1993, 509 women in Ireland died from lung cancer, and smoking is considered to be a major causative factor in almost 90 per cent of deaths from this disease (Department of Health, 1995c). Smoking during pregnancy may have a number of negative consequences for the unborn baby ranging from low birth-weight and reduced intra-uterine growth to foetal loss and spontaneous abortion (Bonati and Fellin, 1991; Bolumar et al., 1994; Tollestrup, Frost and Starzyk, 1992). It has been estimated that babies born to women who smoke weigh approximately 200g less than those born to women who do not smoke (Meredith, 1975). In addition, research has indicated that smoking by parents is a significant contributory factor in the causation of sudden infant deaths (Bergman and Wiesner, 1976). Smoking has also been found to be a significant risk factor for depression in pregnancy (Pritchard, 1994; Hann, Faden and Dufour, 1994; Meyer et al., 1994).

While deaths directly attributable to alcohol are difficult to quantify, the high level of morbidity associated with alcohol abuse is indicated by the fact that about one quarter of admissions to psychiatric hospitals in Ireland are for alcohol-related disorders. Low birth-weight has been found to occur more frequently in women who drink during pregnancy (Lazzaroni et al., 1993). Excessive alcohol consumption during pregnancy may also result in foetal alcohol syndrome, which may damage the unborn baby in a number of ways, including growth retardation, mental retardation, physical malformations and/or pre-term delivery (Daly et al., 1992).

Given the detrimental effects that the use of tobacco and the misuse of substances like alcohol and tranquillisers may have on women's health and on the health of their babies antenatally and postnatally, this part of the study is concerned with an assessment of the level of use of such substances among Irish women. Providing some insight into the level of information prevailing on the risks associated with the use of these substances constitutes an additional objective for this investigation.

With regard to smoking, it is estimated that half the female population in Ireland have never smoked, 29 per cent currently smoke regularly and 16 per cent consider themselves to be ex-smokers. These estimates are consistent with the results of previous research on the smoking behaviour of women in Ireland (Irish Heart Foundation, 1994). Two-thirds of women who smoke would like to give up smoking, while a quarter would choose not to stop smoking. Almost two-thirds (63 per cent) of mothers who smoke are estimated to have continued smoking during pregnancy. With regard to future pregnancies, an estimated 23 per cent of women smokers of child-bearing age indicate that they would continue to smoke. When questioned about the relationship between smoking and specific risk factors, over 90 per cent of women correctly agreed that smoking increases the risk of lung cancer, heart disease and bronchitis. While an estimated 73 per cent correctly agreed that smoking by pregnant women results in the unborn baby smoking too, it is cause for concern that 27 per cent either disagreed with this statement or did not know the correct answer. It is worrying that one woman in every four does not know that smoking increases the risk of narrowing of the arteries.

Close to 77 per cent of women take a drink, while 21 per cent have never taken alcohol. For 47 per cent, beer is the most commonly consumed alcohol followed by spirits at 30 per cent and wine at 20 per cent. Three-quarters of women drink between two and four drinks at any one time. Close to 56 per cent of women say that they have not been intoxicated in the previous 12 months, while 21 per cent say that they have been intoxicated once or twice, with 11 per cent intoxicated between three and five times. Almost half the female population say that they drink to be sociable while 29 per cent enjoy a drink and 19 per cent drink to relax. During pregnancy, one in every two maternal drinkers gave up drink, while one in every five continued drinking as usual. For a future pregnancy, 58 per cent of women drinkers of child-bearing age say that they would give up drink, while 12 per cent indicate that they would continue drinking as usual.

Of the 15 per cent of women estimated to have taken tranquillisers to cope with stress, 42 per cent are estimated to have taken them for more than three months, 31 per cent for one to three months and a quarter for less than one month. The sources of stress vary widely, with family bereavement and marital/relationship problems being specified by a high proportion of women. The most frequently mentioned approaches to coping with a stressful event include talking to family/partner, talking to friends and praying.

More detailed analyses of the factors associated with the use of these substances will be presented in the following sections.

Smoking Behaviour

It is probably not surprising that experience with smoking is significantly related to age. Smoking behaviour by age group is presented in Table 2.1. For women aged 18–30, and 40–50, it has been estimated that about 30 per cent smoke regularly. At 34 per cent, the 30–34-year-old group of women constitutes the highest proportion of regular smokers. A low of one-fifth is estimated for those aged between 55 and 60. The proportion of women who have never smoked varies between 45 and 55 per cent for all age groups. At about 55 per cent, the estimated proportion of women who have never smoked is highest in the youngest and oldest age groups. A low of 45 per cent of non-smokers is estimated for those aged 40–44.

Smoking behaviour is significantly related to social class. Table 2.2 shows that the differences between the non-manual and the manual classes are particularly striking. While over half of the women in the non-manual classes never smoked, this drops below 40 per cent for women in the manual classes. At 16 per cent, the proportion of regular smokers is smallest for women in the higher

Table 2.1: Experience with Smoking and Taking Tranquillisers, by Age Group

Age Group*	Smoking Behaviour*				Ever Taken Tranquillisers?*	
	Smoke Regularly	Smoke Occasionally	Ex-Smoker	Never Smoked	Yes	No
	%	%	%	%	%	%
18–24	29.5	8.1	7.8	54.7	3.3	96.8
25–29	30.0	7.5	12.5	50.0	8.7	91.3
30–34	33.5	5.5	14.5	46.5	10.6	89.4
35–39	27.3	4.9	21.3	46.6	11.2	88.8
40–44	29.2	5.0	20.8	45.1	19.5	80.5
45–49	30.9	4.1	18.7	46.3	21.7	78.3
50–54	29.6	5.7	16.6	48.1	29.2	70.8
55–60	21.1	2.5	20.8	55.6	30.6	69.4
All	29.1	5.7	15.8	49.4	14.8	85.2

* $p < 0.001$.

professional class, with this proportion increasing to over 40 per cent for women in the manual classes. Table 2.2 also shows that 38 per cent of women with medical cards are estimated to smoke regularly, with the corresponding proportion for non-medical-card holders estimated at 26 per cent. Women without medical cards are more likely never to have smoked.

Smoking behaviour by educational experience, employment status and geographical location is presented in Table 2.3. The proportion of women estimated to smoke regularly decreases with increasing levels of education from a high of 41 per cent for those with primary education to a low of 10 per cent for women with university qualifications. The proportion of women who have never smoked increases from 40 per cent at the primary level to 68 per cent for those with university education. At 40 per cent, unemployed women have the highest proportion of smokers relative to other categories of employment. The group including students, the retired, the ill/disabled, together with women working

Table 2.2: Experience with Smoking and Taking Tranquillisers, by Social Class and Medical-Card Status

	Smoking Behaviour*				Ever Taken Tranquillisers?*	
	Smoke Regularly	Smoke Occasionally	Ex-Smoker	Never Smoked	Yes	No
Social Class*	%	%	%	%	%	%
Higher Professional	15.8	6.1	23.6	54.4	14.1	85.9
Lower Professional	21.8	3.8	21.0	53.4	13.3	86.7
Other Non-Manual	25.5	5.9	15.2	53.5	13.5	86.5
Skilled Manual	40.0	4.7	15.7	39.6	22.0	78.0
Semi-Skilled Manual	40.9	6.4	13.0	39.7	15.9	84.1
Unskilled Manual	41.2	6.6	14.0	38.2	19.4	80.6
All	29.9	5.9	16.8	48.0	15.5	84.5
Medical-Card Status*						
Yes	37.6	5.4	14.3	42.6	21.9	78.1
No	25.7	5.6	16.5	52.2	11.8	88.2
All	29.3	5.5	15.8	49.3	14.8	85.2

* $p < 0.001$.

full-time, has the highest proportion of women who never smoked. While one-third of urban women are regular smokers, this contrasts with less than a quarter of rural women who fall into this category.

Whether or not women would like to give up smoking is significantly related to age. Table 2.4 shows that while 81 per cent of women smokers aged between 30 and 34 would like to give up smoking, this contrasts with the estimate of 53 per cent for women in the 55–60 age group. Irrespective of medical-card status, educational experience or geographical location, it is estimated that

Table 2.3: Smoking Behaviour and Ever Taken Tranquillisers, by Education Level, Employment Status and Geographical Location

	Smoking Behaviour				Ever Taken Tranquillisers?	
	Smoke Regularly	Smoke Occasionally	Ex-Smoker	Never Smoked	Yes	No
Education Level*	%	%	%	%	%	%
Primary Cert/Lower	40.9	3.3	15.7	40.0	26.1	73.9
Inter/Group/ Junior Cert	33.0	7.1	16.9	42.9	15.3	84.7
Leaving Cert/ Matric	24.7	5.4	15.7	54.2	9.7	90.4
Qualification from RTC etc.	23.6	7.4	11.6	57.4	7.3	92.7
University Qualification	10.0	6.3	16.0	67.7	12.6	87.4
All	29.2	5.5	15.8	49.4	14.8	85.2
Employment Status*						
Working Full-time	25.3	6.1	14.3	54.4	8.5	91.5
Working Part-time	32.5	4.3	19.3	43.9	17.3	82.7
Unemployed	40.3	5.4	7.1	47.3	7.6	92.4
Home Duties	31.3	4.9	18.7	45.2	21.3	78.7
Student/ Retired/Ill/ Disabled	22.9	10.0	8.9	58.2	6.6	93.4
All	29.2	5.5	15.8	49.4	14.8	85.2
Geographical Location**						
Rural	23.2	7.2	17.7	52.0	12.3	87.8
Urban	32.9	4.7	14.6	47.8	16.5	83.5
All	29.1	5.7	15.8	49.4	14.8	85.2

*   p < 0.001.
** Geographical location by smoking behaviour: p < 0.001.
      Geographical location by taken tranquillisers?: p < 0.005.

between 60 and 70 per cent of women would like to give up smoking. Having had a baby is significantly related to wanting to give up smoking. Close to 71 per cent of women who have had a baby would like to give up smoking, compared with an estimate of 60 per cent for women who have not had a baby.

Table 2.4: Like to Give Up Smoking by Age Group[†]

Age Group*	Like to Give up Smoking?		
	Yes %	No %	Don't Know %
18–24	60.8	27.3	11.9
25–29	65.2	30.0	4.8
30–34	80.6	16.8	2.7
35–39	69.7	25.5	4.8
40–44	75.3	21.1	3.6
45–49	61.1	26.8	12.1
50–54	66.2	27.7	6.1
55–60	53.3	44.2	2.5
All	67.2	26.3	6.5

* $p < 0.001$.
† Analysis based on 1,040 (34.9 per cent) women in the sample who smoke regularly or occasionally.

Smoking behaviour of Irish women during pregnancy was analysed in more detail for women who smoke, and the results are presented in Tables 2.5, 2.6, 2.7, 2.8 and 2.9. An earlier study of a population of pregnant women attending an Irish maternity hospital found that 63 per cent smoked prior to pregnancy and just 5 per cent stopped smoking during pregnancy (Daly, Kiely, Clarke and Matthews, 1992). This contrasts with the results of a Spanish study of pregnant women which found that while 60 per cent of women smoked prior to pregnancy, 48 per cent stopped smoking during pregnancy (Bolumar et al., 1994). While a number of Swedish studies have found that around 30 per cent of women were smokers at the start of their pregnancy, Cnattingius, Lindmark and Meirik (1992) estimated that 29 per cent of these stopped smoking at some stage during the pregnancy, while Lindqvist and Aberg (1992) estimated that 18 per cent continued to smoke while pregnant.

While age and medical-card status were not significantly related to smoking behaviour during a previous pregnancy, these
variables did have a significant effect on the intention to smoke
during a future pregnancy. Table 2.5 indicates that between 20
and 30 per cent of women smokers aged between 25 and 49 years
would expect to smoke during a future pregnancy; the estimate
for those planning not to smoke ranges between 60 and 70 per
cent for the same age group. While medical-card status was not
significantly related to having smoked during a previous pregnancy,
one-third of women smokers with medical cards indicate that they
would continue smoking during a future pregnancy. Overall, 50
per cent of women smokers with medical cards indicate that they
would not smoke during a future pregnancy, compared with approximately two out of every three non-medical-card holders.

**Table 2.5: Intention to Smoke During a Future Pregnancy,
by Age Group and Medical-Card Status**

	Intention to Smoke During a Future Pregnancy[†]		
	Yes	*No*	*Don't Know*
Age Group*	*%*	*%*	*%*
18–24	13.8	68.8	17.4
25–29	25.5	64.2	10.4
30–34	26.7	60.0	12.8
35–39	21.8	67.2	11.1
40–44	28.2	62.6	9.3
45–49	22.7	61.7	15.7
All	22.6	64.4	12.9
Medical-Card Status**			
Yes	32.5	53.6	13.9
No	18.7	68.4	12.9
All	23.0	63.7	13.2

* $p < 0.01$.

** $p < 0.001$.

†   Analysis by age group limited to the 1,179 (39.6 per cent) women of child-
     bearing age in the sample who have smoked.

     Analysis by medical-card status limited to the 1,146 (39.8 per cent)
     women of child-bearing age in the sample who have smoked for whom
     medical-card status is available.

Table 2.6 shows that the proportion of mothers who smoked during a previous pregnancy decreases with increasing levels of education. This finding is consistent with the research results of other studies on this question (Fingerhut et al., 1990; Clissold, Hopkins and Desson, 1991; Berman and Gritz, 1991; Abma and Mott, 1991; Brosky, 1995). The highest estimate of 72 per cent is found for mothers with primary education compared with a low of 39 per cent for mothers with university qualifications. While the estimated proportion of women at the primary level who would smoke during a future pregnancy drops to 31 per cent, there is a smaller decrease to 17 per cent for those with university education. The estimation of a logistic regression model for mothers who smoked during pregnancy found that the social class effect was confounded within level of education. Having controlled for this confounding, the probability of maternal smokers having smoked during a previous pregnancy was estimated at the high level of 72 per cent for women with primary education only compared with 31 per cent for those with third-level education.

Employment status has a significant effect on smoking behaviour during a previous pregnancy and the intention to smoke during a future pregnancy. Table 2.6 shows that while 90 per cent of unemployed women smokers continued smoking during a previous pregnancy, one in every three women in this group indicate that they would continue to smoke during a future pregnancy. Even though one in every two women smokers working part-time continued to smoke during pregnancy, this is the lowest proportion for any employment group. Over 70 per cent of working-women smokers say that they would not smoke during a future pregnancy, compared with just over half the group of unemployed women smokers. Table 2.6 also shows that urban mothers who smoke are more likely to have continued to smoke during a previous pregnancy, while a higher proportion of rural women smokers would give up smoking during a future pregnancy.

Social class has a significant effect on whether or not women smokers intend to smoke during a future pregnancy. Table 2.7 shows that even though between a half and three-quarters of women across all social groups say that they would not smoke during a future pregnancy, there is a clear class effect in evidence for those who would choose to smoke. The proportion of women in all of the manual classes who would choose to smoke

Table 2.6: Smoked During a Previous Pregnancy[†] and Intention to Smoke During a Future Pregnancy,[††] by Education Level, Employment Status and Geographical Location, for Women who Smoke

	Smoked During a Previous Pregnancy			Intention to Smoke During a Future Pregnancy		
	Yes	No	Can't Remember	Yes	No	Don't Know
Education Level*	%	%	%	%	%	%
Primary Cert/Lower	71.8	27.7	0.4	31.4	54.0	14.7
Inter/Group/Junior Cert.	63.4	36.3	0.3	25.6	59.9	14.6
Leaving Cert/Matric.	56.5	42.9	0.6	18.1	69.2	12.7
Qualification from RTC etc.	46.8	53.2	0.0	7.9	80.5	11.7
University Qualification	39.4	58.9	1.8	16.9	83.1	0.0
All	62.8	36.8	0.5	22.5	64.5	13.0
Employment Status**						
Working Full-time	60.1	39.4	0.5	15.4	71.0	13.6
Working Part-time	51.8	46.6	1.6	16.3	70.1	13.7
Unemployed	89.8	10.2	0.0	34.9	50.4	14.7
Home Duties	63.0	36.7	0.4	28.8	59.7	11.6
Student/Retired/Ill/Disabled	75.6	24.4	0.0	12.0	71.4	16.7
All	62.7	36.8	0.5	22.6	64.4	12.9
Geographical Location***						
Rural	51.9	41.8	0.3	18.0	72.5	9.5
Urban	65.7	33.7	0.6	25.1	60.1	14.8
All	62.7	36.8	0.5	22.6	64.4	12.9

*   p < 0.001.

**   Employment status by "smoked during a previous pregnancy": p < 0.01.
       Employment status by "intention to smoke during a future pregnancy":
       p < 0.001.

***   Geographical location by "smoked during a previous pregnancy": p <0.05.
       Geographical location by "intention to smoke during a future pregnancy": p < 0.001.

†   Analysis by education level limited to the 1,056 (35.9 per cent) maternal smokers in the sample for whom education level attained is available.
       Analysis by employment status and geographical location limited to the 1,063 (35.7 per cent) maternal smokers in the sample.

††   Analysis by education level limited to the 1,170 (39.7 per cent) women of child-bearing age in the sample who have smoked and for whom education level attained is available.
       Analysis by employment status and geographical location limited to the 1,179 (39.6 per cent) women of child-bearing age in the sample who have smoked.

during a future pregnancy is substantially more than that estimated for any of the professional or non-manual classes. It is
particularly interesting that almost one in four women in the unskilled manual class answered "don't know" when asked whether
or not they would smoke during a future pregnancy. In an American study during the late 1980s, Milham and Davis (1991) also
found a relationship between smoking prevalence during pregnancy and social class. A logistic regression analysis undertaken
by King, Barry and Carter (1993) found that socioeconomic status
was a strong predictor of smoking status in the US as women at
the lower socioeconomic level were 3.7 times more likely to smoke
during pregnancy than those in higher socioeconomic classes.

**Table 2.7: Intention to Smoke During a Future Pregnancy
Distributed by Social Class[†]**

	Intention to Smoke During a Future Pregnancy[†]		
	Yes	*No*	*Don't Know*
*Social Class**[*]	*%*	*%*	*%*
Higher Professional	17.9	76.2	5.9
Lower Professional	18.8	70.9	10.3
Other Non-Manual	18.3	69.4	12.3
Skilled Manual	32.3	56.4	11.3
Semi-Skilled Manual	31.1	55.2	13.7
Unskilled Manual	19.1	57.7	23.1
All	23.5	64.1	12.5

[*] $p < 0.001$.

[†] Analysis limited to the 1,112 (40.8 per cent) women of child-bearing age
who have smoked and for whom social class is known.

In attempting to assess the multivariate effect on intention to
smoke during future pregnancies for women and mothers, logistic
regression models were estimated for both groups. The results of
the logistic regression analysis for women smokers' intentions
during a future pregnancy are presented in Table A1 in Appendix
3 and show that:

• Women smokers are more likely to say that they would not
  smoke during a future pregnancy.

- Women smokers with medical cards, unemployed women and urban residents are more likely than non-medical-card holders, women in other employment categories, and rural residents, to say that they would smoke during a future pregnancy.

To illustrate the effect of these results on the probability of smoking during a future pregnancy, Table 2.8 presents predicted probabilities for women smokers with specific characteristics. The 12 per cent of working-women smokers living in a rural area without a medical card who say that they would smoke during a future pregnancy contrasts sharply with the estimate of 51 per cent for urban, unemployed women smokers with medical cards.

Table 2.8: Estimated Percentages of Women Smokers of Child-bearing Age who would Smoke During a Future Pregnancy, with Characteristics Defined According to Medical-Card Status, Employment Status and Area of Residence

	Would Smoke During a Future Pregnancy %

Living in a Rural Area
    Working Full-time
    No Medical Card
	12

Living in a Rural Area
    Unemployed
    No Medical Card
	27

Living in an Urban Area
    Unemployed
    No Medical Card
	39

Living in an Urban Area
    Unemployed
    With Medical Card
	51

The parameter estimates for the logistic regression model fitted for whether or not maternal smokers would smoke during a future pregnancy are presented in Table A2, Appendix 3. Medical-card status, area of residence and whether or not smoking was continued during a previous pregnancy proved to be significant in this model and indicate that:

- Mothers who smoke are more likely to say that they would not smoke during a future pregnancy.

- Relative to rural maternal smokers and non-medical-card holders, urban maternal smokers and those with medical cards are more likely to say that they would smoke during a future pregnancy.

- Relative to those who did not smoke during a previous pregnancy, women who have smoked during previous pregnancies are more likely to smoke during future pregnancies.

To illustrate the effect of these results on the probability of smoking during a future pregnancy, Table 2.9 presents predicted probabilities for maternal smokers with specific characteristics. Only 3 per cent of rural maternal smokers, without medical cards who did not smoke during a previous pregnancy would be expected to smoke during a future pregnancy. This compares with the estimate of 61 per cent for urban maternal smokers, with medical cards who did smoke during a previous pregnancy.

Table 2.9: Estimated Percentages of Maternal Smokers of Child-bearing Age who would Smoke During a Future Pregnancy, with Characteristics Defined According to Medical-Card Status, Area of Residence and Whether They Smoked During a Previous Pregnancy

		Percentage who Would Smoke During a Future Pregnancy	
		Previous Pregnancies	
		Smoked	*Did Not Smoke*
Geographical Location	*Medical-Card Status*	*%*	*%*
Rural	Yes	49	5
	No	36	3
Urban	Yes	61	7
	No	48	4

Consumption of Alcohol

From the survey results, it is estimated that 77 per cent of Irish women take a drink, and Table 2.10 shows that this varies by age

and medical-card status. Over 80 per cent of women aged between
25 and 40 years take a drink, compared with 60 per cent of those
aged 55–60. Over 30 per cent of women aged 50 and over have
never taken alcohol, compared with an estimate of less than 20
per cent for those aged under 45 years. The estimates by medical-
card status are also interesting, with 27 per cent of medical-card
holders never having taken alcohol, compared with 18 per cent of
non-medical-card holders. At 80 per cent, a higher proportion of
women without medical cards drink than do medical-card holders
(69 per cent).

**Table 2.10: Consumption of Alcohol, by Age Group and
Medical-Card Status**

	Consumption of Alcohol		
	Takes a Drink	*Ex-Drinker*	*Never Drinks*
Age Group*	%	%	%
18–24	79.7	1.0	19.3
25–29	81.7	2.9	15.4
30–34	82.7	2.2	15.1
35–39	81.8	3.9	14.3
40–44	79.7	3.9	16.5
45–49	74.9	2.3	22.8
50–54	65.1	2.8	32.1
55–60	60.0	2.0	38.0
All	76.9	2.5	20.5
Medical-Card Status*			
Yes	69.1	4.3	26.6
No	80.4	1.8	17.8
All	77.0	2.5	20.5

* p < 0.001.

Table 2.11 shows that the probability of taking a drink increases
with increasing levels of education, with an estimate of 70 per cent
presented for women with primary education only, compared with
84 per cent for those with university qualifications. At 27 per cent,
the highest estimate for women who have never taken alcohol is

found for those at the primary level. It is also evident from Table 2.11 that working women are more likely to drink than those engaged in home duties. Almost one in four women engaged in home duties has never taken a drink. The proportion of women in rural areas who have never taken a drink is close to 30 per cent, while 83 per cent of women in urban areas take a drink regularly.

Table 2.11: Consumption of Alcohol, by Education Level, Employment Status and Geographical Location

	Consumption of Alcohol		
	Takes a Drink	*Ex-Drinker*	*Never Drinks*
*Education Level**	%	%	%
Primary Cert/Lower	69.8	3.4	26.8
Inter/Group/Junior Cert	75.6	3.0	21.5
Leaving Cert/Matric	80.6	1.8	17.6
Qualification from RTC etc.	78.3	1.9	19.8
University Qualification	83.8	2.2	14.0
All	77.1	2.5	20.4
*Employment Status**			
Working Full-time	81.2	2.2	16.6
Working Part-time	84.6	2.3	13.1
Unemployed	77.8	4.5	17.7
Home Duties	73.2	3.1	23.8
Student/Retired/Ill/ Disabled	74.5	0.0	25.5
All	76.9	2.5	20.5
*Geographical Location**			
Rural	68.0	2.3	29.8
Urban	82.7	2.7	14.6
All	76.9	2.5	20.5

* $p < 0.001$.

Estimates for the consumption of alcohol during a previous pregnancy, together with expectations regarding the consumption of alcohol during a future pregnancy, are presented by age group and medical-card status, where relevant, in Table 2.12. Between age

30 and 49 years an increasing proportion of mothers are estimated to have given up drinking during a previous pregnancy,

**Table 2.12: Consumption of Alcohol During a Previous
Pregnancy[†] and Intentions Regarding Consumption of
Alcohol During a Future Pregnancy,[††] by Age Group and
Medical-Card Status, where significant**

Age Group*	Consumption of Alcohol During a Previous Pregnancy			Intention to Consume Alcohol During a Future Pregnancy		
	Continued drinking as usual	Cut down	Gave up drinking	Continue drinking as usual	Cut down	Give up drinking
	%	%	%	%	%	%
18–24	15.1	19.4	65.5	5.3	31.7	63.1
25–29	17.0	28.1	54.9	8.5	29.6	61.9
30–34	15.7	40.2	44.1	12.4	33.3	54.3
35–39	19.1	33.1	47.8	18.3	30.6	51.1
40–44	22.9	29.1	48.0	16.5	30.7	52.8
45–49	26.0	21.1	52.9	20.8	21.8	57.5
50–54	29.6	20.9	49.5	—	—	—
55–60	24.1	14.0	61.9	—	—	—
All	21.3	27.9	50.8	12.1	30.4	57.6
Medical-Card Status*						
Yes				17.0	29.0	54.1
No				10.3	30.8	58.9
All				12.0	30.3	57.7

* $p < 0.001$.

†   Analysis by age group limited to the 1,526 (51.2 per cent) mothers in the sample who drink.

†† Analysis by age group limited to the 1,707 (57.3 per cent) women of child-bearing age in the sample who drink.

Analysis by medical-card status limited to the 1,651 (57.3 per cent) women of child-bearing age in the sample who drink and for whom medical-card status is available.

with over half of all mothers across all age groups found in this category. The proportion of women who say that they would continue drinking as usual during a future pregnancy increases with age and reaches a high of 21 per cent for those in the 45–49 age group. The trends in evidence here are consistent with the results of a previous Irish study which found that 66 per cent of pregnant women reduced their alcohol consumption, while 11 per cent gave up alcohol completely while pregnant (Daly, Kiely, Clarke, Matthews, 1992). These Irish results contrast with those reported by a study of Spanish women which found that 37 per cent of pregnant women drinkers stopped consuming alcohol while pregnant (Bolumar et al., 1994).

Medical-card status was not significantly related to drinking history during previous pregnancies, though there was a significant effect on the declared intention to drink alcohol during a future pregnancy. While 17 per cent of women medical-card holders would be expected to continue drinking as usual during a future pregnancy, irrespective of medical-card status, over half the women of child-bearing age would be expected to give up drinking during a future pregnancy.

Table 2.13 shows drinking behaviour during previous pregnancies and anticipated drinking behaviour during future pregnancies by education level and employment status, where significant. While drinking history during a previous pregnancy was not significantly related to education, the proportion of women estimated to continue drinking as usual during a future pregnancy decreases with increasing levels of education. One woman in five with primary education says that she would continue to drink during a future pregnancy compared with 7 per cent for women with university qualifications. Close to 24 per cent of mothers engaged in home duties continued to drink during pregnancy, compared with 9 per cent of unemployed mothers, while close to one in every two women in both groups gave up drinking when pregnant. The number of women drinkers who would give up drink during a future pregnancy is estimated at between 50 and 70 per cent across all categories of employment.

A logistic regression analysis of the intentions of mothers regarding drinking during a future pregnancy found that drinking behaviour during a prior pregnancy was the only significant predictor of future behaviour: women who had continued drinking

Table 2.13: Consumption of Alcohol During a Previous Pregnancy[†] and Intentions Regarding Consumption of Alcohol During a Future Pregnancy,[††] by Education Level and Employment Status, where significant

	Consumption of Alcohol During a Previous Pregnancy			Consumption of Alcohol During a Future Pregnancy		
	Continued drinking as usual	Cut down	Gave up drinking	Continue drinking as usual	Cut down	Give up drinking
*Education Level**	%	%	%	%	%	%
Primary Cert/Lower				20.2	27.7	52.2
Inter/Group/Junior Cert				12.8	28.4	58.8
Leaving Cert/Matric				10.2	32.1	57.7
Qualification from RTC etc.				11.1	34.7	54.2
University Qualification				6.5	28.1	65.4
All				12.0	30.3	57.7
*Employment Status***						
Working Full-time	17.5	31.4	51.1	8.2	33.0	58.7
Working Part-time	18.4	27.5	54.1	14.9	25.1	60.0
Unemployed	8.9	42.5	48.6	10.8	22.8	66.5
Home Duties	23.7	26.0	50.3	17.8	29.9	52.3
Student/Retired/ Ill/Disabled	12.6	30.7	56.8	3.9	29.6	66.5
All	21.3	27.9	50.8	12.1	30.4	57.6

* $P < 0.001$.

**   Employment status by "consumption of alcohol during a previous pregnancy": $p < 0.05$.
       Employment status by "consumption of alcohol during a future pregnancy": $p < 0.001$.

†   Analysis by employment status limited to the 1,526 (51.2 per cent) mothers in the sample who drink.

††   Analysis by education level limited to the 1,692 (57.5 per cent) women of child-bearing age in the sample who drink and for whom education level attained is available.
       Analysis by employment status limited to the 1,707 (57.3 per cent) women of child-bearing age in the sample who drink.

during a previous pregnancy would be more likely to continue to drink during a future pregnancy. A logistic regression model was also estimated for whether women of child-bearing age who drink would continue to drink during a future pregnancy. This analysis found that age was insignificant and that education and medical-card status were confounded by whether or not the women was a mother. The parameter estimates for this analysis are presented in Table A3 in Appendix 3 and the results indicate that:

- Relative to mothers, women who have never had a baby are more likely to give up drinking during a future pregnancy.

- Women on home duties are most likely to continue drinking as usual while those working full-time are least likely to continue drinking as usual during a future pregnancy.

An illustration of the effect of these results is presented in Table 2.14. While only 6 per cent of women working full-time having their first baby would expect to continue drinking as usual during a future pregnancy, this estimate increases to a high of 18 per cent for mothers engaged in home duties. Approximately two out of every three first time mothers, working part-time would expect to give up drink during a future pregnancy.

Table 2.14: Estimated Percentages for Women of Child-bearing Age who Drink, with Regard to Their Drinking Intentions During a Future Pregnancy

	Women of Child-bearing Age who Drink:		
	Drinking Intentions During a Future Pregnancy		
	Continue as Usual	*Cut Down*	*Give Up*
	%	%	%
Mother Working Full-time	11	36	53
Mother Working Part-time	17	25	58
Mother on Home Duties	18	30	51
Working Full-time, Not a Mother	6	32	62
Working Part-time, Not a Mother	9	23	68

Use of Tranquillisers

Whether or not tranquillisers had been taken to help cope with
stress is presented by age group in Table 2.1. There is a clear age
relationship in evidence here, with the proportion of women estimated to have taken tranquillisers under stress increasing from 3
per cent for the 18–24 year olds to around 20 per cent for the 40–
50 group, with a high of around 30 per cent estimated for those
aged between 50 and 60. It should be noted, however, that the approach to prescribing and taking tranquillisers may have changed
over time and this may, to some extent, be reflected in the age effect in evidence here. The proportion of women with medical cards
who are estimated to have taken tranquillisers is shown in Table
2.2 to be substantially greater when compared with other women.
While more than one-fifth of women medical-card holders are estimated to have taken tranquillisers to help cope with stress, the
corresponding figure for non-medical-card holders is 12 per cent.

Table 2.3 shows that 26 per cent of women with primary education used tranquillisers at some time, compared with 13 per
cent of women with university qualifications. Women engaged in
home duties and those working part-time were also more likely to
have taken tranquillisers, with estimates of 21 per cent and 17
per cent, respectively. With an estimate of 17 per cent, women in
urban areas were somewhat more likely to have taken tranquillisers than women in rural areas with an estimate of 12 per cent.
It is worth noting that close to a fifth of married women and those
who have had a baby have taken tranquillisers at some time,
compared with an estimate of around 7 per cent for single women
and those who have not had children.

Conclusion

Despite clear and consistent evidence of the health risks associated with smoking, an estimated 29 per cent of Irish women
smoke regularly. In addition to the personal health risks incurred,
smoking during pregnancy has adverse effects on the birth outcome. It is therefore cause for serious concern that despite these
risks, 63 per cent of women who smoke continued to smoke while
pregnant, and close to 25 per cent of women smokers of child-
bearing age said that they would smoke during a future pregnancy. These findings must raise serious questions about the ef-

fectiveness of current policies aimed at encouraging the pursuit of healthier lifestyles by Irish women. This concern is supported by the finding that only 58 per cent of women of child-bearing age would plan on giving up drinking during a future pregnancy.

While these issues do feature in the Department of Health's Health Promotion Strategy (1995c), the action proposed is broadly specified as "encouraging the avoidance of smoking and alcohol and drug misuse before and during pregnancy" (p. 20). A review of the literature on this subject would indicate, however, that targeted, strategic programmes are required if smoking and alcohol misuse by women in general, and pregnant women in particular, is to be successfully addressed. While Howell (1994) called for a total ban on all tobacco advertising, a number of studies have shown some success for mass media campaigns which highlight the risks of smoking and alcohol consumption during pregnancy (Campion et al., 1994; Casiro et al., 1994). Studies from two Nordic countries found that specifically designed intervention programmes aimed at assisting pregnant women in stopping smoking helped to motivate more women to stop smoking (Valbo and Nylander, 1994; Haug, Aaro and Fugelli, 1994). However, as less well educated and younger women are less likely to receive early prenatal care, the challenge of achieving a reduction in smoking prevalence amongst these women must not be underestimated (Abma and Mott, 1991).

In their study of pregnant women attending an Irish maternity hospital, Daly, Kiely, Clarke and Matthews (1992) found that while 57 per cent of respondents said that a doctor had told them that smoking while pregnant was harmful to the baby, only 11 per cent said that a doctor had told them about the danger to the baby of continued alcohol consumption. This finding led these authors to the conclusion that "it is necessary to educate and convince doctors of the benefits of reducing alcohol intake in pregnancy" (p. 157). This recommendation is supported by other studies which found a positive benefit from systematic intervention by physicians and other health professionals in smoking cessation programmes and the promotion of healthier lifestyles for pregnant women (Brosky, 1995; Clissold, Hopkins and Seddon, 1991).

The substantial and positive effects that might be expected from a reduction in smoking by pregnant women may be indicated by the estimation for the United States that if all women stopped smoking when pregnant, peri-natal mortality rates would fall by

approximately 10 per cent (Kleinman et al., 1988). It has been
proposed that the comprehensive strategies necessary to achieve
a reduction in smoking and alcohol consumption should include
the basic components of research, outreach, education and advocacy (*Health Objectives for the Nation*, 1994). Despite the risks to
their own health and to that of their unborn babies, too many
Irish women smoke both during and outside pregnancy and too
many women continue to drink while pregnant. If the health
needs of these women are to be truly addressed, the research
findings presented here indicate that these basic components
should be considered an essential part of future strategies aimed
at reducing smoking and alcohol consumption among Irish
women.

3

Sex Education

Introduction

In the national survey of health needs, women were asked questions about their experience of sex education and the risk factors associated with infection with the AIDS virus. One of the concerns being addressed here was whether the receipt of formal sex education was becoming more the norm for Irish women. In addition, it was considered important to assess the level of understanding prevailing regarding the risks to which women may become exposed, including pregnancy and the AIDS virus.

Overall, 49 per cent of women received sex education while growing up, with the majority receiving information in school and/ or from parents/guardians. While 64 per cent considered the sex education received to be adequate, for 36 per cent it was inadequate/very inadequate. With regard to the risk of pregnancy under specific conditions, the majority of women know that it is possible to become pregnant while breast-feeding, while having sexual intercourse for the first time and while going through the menopause. Close to three out of four women know that a woman is most likely to become pregnant in the middle of her cycle. This means, however, that one in every four women does not know when she is most at risk of pregnancy. Experience of sex education and the understanding of when a woman is at risk of pregnancy were found to be significantly influenced by demographic factors and these are discussed in more detail in the next section.

Demographic Effects on Experience of Sex Education

Table 3.1 shows that age is significantly associated with whether or not sex education was received, where it was received and whether it was perceived to be adequate. The trend in the relationship between these variables is also evident from this table. The proportion of each age group reporting that they had received sex education declines from a high of 88 per cent for the 18–24 age group to a low of 15 per cent for the 55–60 age group. While a majority of the 18–24 group received sex education in school, this estimate declines over the age groups to a low of 27 per cent for the 55–60-year-olds. The perception of adequacy also declines from the younger age groups to the older groups with three-quarters of the youngest age group considering the sex education received to be adequate. The corresponding estimate is just less than half for the 55–60 age group.

Table 3.1: Receipt, Location and Adequacy of Sex Education Received, by Age Group

Age Group	Sex Education Received*		Where Sex Education Received*[†]			Adequacy of Sex Education*[†]	
	Yes	*No*	*School*	*Parents*	*Other*	*Adequate*	*Inadequate*
	%	%	%	%	%	%	%
18–24	87.8	12.2	54.0	38.4	7.7	74.5	25.5
25–29	70.1	29.9	53.2	38.7	8.1	65.8	34.2
30–34	53.2	46.8	49.3	40.9	9.9	56.0	44.0
35–39	44.9	55.1	46.6	46.0	7.4	53.8	46.2
40–44	34.9	65.1	39.7	50.5	9.9	51.9	48.1
45–49	20.5	79.5	28.8	59.8	11.4	58.1	41.9
50–54	17.3	82.7	40.0	49.4	10.6	59.9	40.1
55–60	14.7	85.3	27.4	57.8	14.7	49.2	50.8
All	48.5	51.5	49.3	42.1	8.6	63.5	36.5

* $p < 0.001$.
†   Analysis based on 1,449 (48.7 per cent) women in sample who had received sex education.

Information regarding risk of pregnancy by age group is presented in Table 3.2. While 84 per cent of the 35–39 age group know that a woman can get pregnant while breast-feeding, this estimate falls to between 65 and 70 per cent for the 18–24-year-

Table 3.2: Perceived Risk of Pregnancy, by Age Group

	Age Group								
	18–24	*25–29*	*30–34*	*35–39*	*40–44*	*45–49*	*50–54*	*55–60*	*All*
	%	%	%	%	%	%	%	%	%
Cannot get pregnant while breast-feeding*									
Agree	10.6	5.5	8.0	6.2	8.1	8.8	14.3	12.4	9.0
Disagree†	66.1	77.6	81.9	84.1	80.4	74.1	68.5	65.3	74.8
Don't know	23.3	16.9	10.0	9.7	11.5	17.2	17.2	22.4	16.2
Cannot get pregnant during first intercourse*									
Agree	2.0	2.0	2.3	1.1	2.5	3.4	5.8	3.3	2.6
Disagree†	96.2	94.7	95.9	97.1	93.3	91.9	90.2	89.7	94.1
Don't know	1.8	3.3	1.7	1.8	4.1	4.7	4.0	6.9	3.3
Most likely to get pregnant in first few days after period*									
Agree	26.4	29.2	32.5	25.4	27.4	30.6	35.7	36.1	29.8
Disagree†	55.3	57.9	58.4	64.9	62.0	56.5	46.3	41.7	56.1
Don't know	18.3	12.9	9.1	9.8	10.6	12.9	17.9	22.2	14.1
Cannot get pregnant going through change of life*									
Agree	9.5	4.1	5.1	3.0	2.6	2.5	4.4	5.2	4.9
Disagree†	74.4	84.8	88.7	91.4	92.3	92.6	89.1	87.9	86.6
Don't know	16.1	11.1	6.3	5.6	5.1	4.9	6.5	7.0	8.5
Woman is most likely to become pregnant*									
Beginning of Cycle	12.5	13.9	8.4	7.2	7.3	9.4	10.2	7.8	9.8
Middle of Cycle†	67.0	71.8	78.3	82.6	78.9	72.9	66.2	65.3	73.0
End of Cycle	5.8	6.7	5.1	5.0	4.4	6.6	10.2	8.7	6.3
Don't know	14.8	7.7	8.1	5.3	9.4	11.1	13.4	18.2	10.9

* $p < 0.001$.

†   Most appropriate response.

olds, and those aged between 50 and 60 years old. That a woman can get pregnant during first intercourse is known by at least 90 per cent of women in all age groups. The risk of getting pregnant during the first few days after a period seems to be associated with the greatest degree of uncertainty/ignorance with, on average, just over half the women knowing that this is unlikely. This contrasts with the "change of life" question where more than 80 per cent of those aged over 24 years know that it is possible to get pregnant at this time. While at least two-thirds of women in all age groups know that a woman is most likely to get pregnant in the middle of her cycle, the fact that between one-third and one-quarter of women across the different age groups are estimated not to know this is cause for concern.

The receipt and adequacy of sex education, together with the perceived risk of pregnancy was found to be significantly related to employment status. Table 3.3 shows that those on home duties ranked lowest in terms of the proportion having received sex education and the perceived adequacy of the education received. This is probably not surprising when it is considered that women engaged in home duties on a full-time basis are more likely to be in the older age groups. With the exception of the "other" category, at least three-quarters of the women in the remaining groups responded correctly to the question regarding the risk of pregnancy while breast-feeding. The risk of pregnancy during the change of life was correctly assessed by more than three-quarters of respondents in all categories. It is noteworthy that, at 60 per cent, the unemployed ranked lowest in terms of knowing that a woman is most likely to get pregnant during the middle stage of her cycle.

Education level attained was found to be significantly related to the receipt of sex education and perceived risk of pregnancy, but the relationship with the adequacy of the sex education received was not significant. Table 3.4 shows that the receipt of sex education is positively associated with the level of education attained, with the low estimate of 18 per cent of women with just primary education having received sex education contrasting with estimates of over 70 per cent for women with a third-level qualification. While there was no significant difference by education level in the understanding of the risk of pregnancy when going through the change of life, Table 3.4 shows that the perceived risk of pregnancy under other conditions was clearly related to level of

Table 3.3: Receipt and Adequacy of Sex Education Together with Perceived Risk of Pregnancy, by Employment Status

	Employment Status				
	Work Full-time[1]	Work Part-time	Unemployed	Home Duties	Other[2]
	%	%	%	%	%
*Was sex education received?**					
Yes	64.5	45.1	62.0	29.9	82.8
No	35.5	54.9	38.0	70.1	17.2
Adequacy of sex education[††]*					
Adequate	64.2	58.0	60.9	56.0	80.1
Inadequate	35.8	42.0	39.1	44.0	19.9
Risk of Pregnancy					
*Cannot get pregnant while breast-feeding**					
Disagree[†]	74.2	80.4	78.3	77.2	57.6
Other	25.8	19.6	21.7	22.8	42.4
*Cannot get pregnant during change of life**					
Disagree[†]	83.2	92.7	77.2	91.0	76.6
Other	16.8	7.3	22.8	9.0	23.4
*Most likely to get pregnant at what stage of cycle?**					
Middle[†]	77.0	81.0	60.3	71.5	67.5
Other	13.0	12.5	25.1	17.3	18.8
Don't Know	10.0	6.5	14.6	11.2	13.7

* $p < 0.001$.
1   Includes relative assisting.
2   Includes student/retired/ill/disabled/others not in labour force.
†   Most appropriate response.
†† Analysis based on 1,449 (48.7 per cent) women in the sample who had received sex education.

Table 3.4: Receipt of Sex Education and Perceived Risk of Pregnancy, by Education Level

	Employment Status				
	Primary Cert/Lower	*Inter/Group/ Junior Cert*	*Leaving Cert/Matric*	*Qualification from RTC, etc.*	*University Qualification*
	%	%	%	%	%
*Was sex education received?**					
Yes	17.6	37.6	65.0	76.9	72.4
No	82.4	62.4	34.9	23.1	27.6
Risk of Pregnancy					
*Cannot get pregnant while breast-feeding**					
Agree	10.3	8.0	9.0	8.5	8.1
Disagree†	67.8	74.6	76.9	74.1	86.4
Don't Know	22.0	17.4	14.2	17.4	5.6
*Cannot get pregnant during first intercourse**					
Agree	3.6	3.7	1.6	1.4	0.0
Disagree†	88.8	93.5	96.7	96.7	100.0
Don't know	7.6	2.8	1.8	1.4	0.0
*Most likely to get pregnant in first few days after period**					
Agree	38.8	35.2	24.3	10.4	17.6
Disagree†	41.9	50.6	63.2	67.8	74.4
Don't Know	19.3	14.2	12.5	10.4	8.0
*Woman is most likely to become pregnant**					
Beginning of Cycle	12.3	12.5	6.9	12.2	7.8
Middle of Cycle†	60.8	68.5	79.2	82.4	86.2
End of Cycle	9.6	7.7	4.6	2.1	1.9
Don't Know	17.4	11.3	9.3	3.3	4.1

* $p < 0.001$.

†   Most appropriate response.

educational attainment. For all of these questions, the proportion of women with primary education only answering correctly was lowest with the highest estimate for correct responses found for women with third-level qualifications. It is of particular concern that 17 per cent of women with primary education only do not know when a women is most likely to become pregnant and more than one woman in five does not know if a woman can get pregnant while breast-feeding. It is also somewhat surprising that only between a half and three-quarters of women with second-level education or higher know that a woman is not at greatest risk of pregnancy the first few days after a period.

While medical-card status was confounded within age, employment status and education, social class was significant for receipt of sex education and perceived risk of pregnancy. Table 3.5 shows a strong class effect with more than half the women in the non-manual classes estimated to have received sex education, compared with a low of 26 per cent of women in the skilled manual group. For each of the questions on the perceived risk of pregnancy, the class effect in evidence in Table 3.5 continues to be strong and consistent: for each question, the proportion of women providing the correct information declines from the highest level within the higher professional group to the lowest level within the unskilled manual group.

Women who had ever had a baby were compared with those who had not had a baby. Just over one-third of mothers have received sex education while the equivalent proportion for other women was 75 per cent. What is perhaps particularly interesting in this analysis is that only about one-half of the women in both groups could correctly answer the question on the risk of getting pregnant in the first few days after a period. Mothers are better informed with regard to the risk of pregnancy during the change of life, with 92 per cent of this group knowing the correct answer compared with just 78 per cent of those women who were not mothers.

The perception regarding risk of pregnancy was cross-tabulated against the question of whether or not sex education was received and the results are presented in Table 3.6. While the results for the risk of pregnancy while breast-feeding were not significant, the perception of the risk of pregnancy during first intercourse, in the first few days after a period and during the change of life was found to be significantly related to whether or not sex education has been received while growing up.

Table 3.5: Receipt of Sex Education and Perceived Risk of Pregnancy, by Social Class

	Social Class					
	Higher Prof.	*Lower Prof.*	*Other Non-Manual*	*Skilled Manual*	*Semi-skilled Manual*	*Unskilled Manual*
Was sex education received?						
Yes	57.3	50.9	50.1	26.3	47.6	35.3
No	42.7	49.1	49.9	73.7	52.4	64.7
Risk of Pregnancy						
Cannot get pregnant while breast-feeding*						
Agree	4.3	7.0	9.3	9.2	10.5	7.8
Disagree†	86.7	83.4	75.7	72.0	70.7	66.7
Don't Know	9.0	9.6	15.0	18.8	18.8	25.5
Cannot get pregnant during first intercourse*						
Agree	0.4	1.4	3.0	4.0	3.1	2.7
Disagree†	99.6	97.3	93.8	93.0	92.3	90.2
Don't Know	0.0	1.3	3.2	3.0	4.6	7.1
Most likely to get pregnant in first few days after period*						
Agree	15.6	23.5	29.0	37.7	37.3	38.7
Disagree†	75.2	67.1	58.4	45.4	47.0	43.2
Don't Know	9.2	9.4	12.6	16.9	15.7	18.1
Cannot get pregnant going through change of life*						
Agree	2.7	3.6	4.6	4.6	5.7	5.1
Disagree†	91.1	92.6	85.5	89.5	85.2	83.0
Don't Know	6.2	3.8	9.9	5.8	9.0	11.9
Woman is most likely to become pregnant*						
Beginning of Cycle	5.3	6.5	9.3	11.6	11.8	13.5
Middle of Cycle†	85.8	83.7	75.2	66.8	66.5	58.6
End of Cycle	2.2	4.3	4.6	9.9	9.6	8.3
Don't Know	6.7	5.4	10.9	11.8	12.1	19.6

* $p < 0.001$.
†   Most appropriate response.

Table 3.6: Perceived Risk of Pregnancy, by Receipt of Sex Education

	Sex Education Received?	
	Yes	No
	%	%
Cannot get pregnant during first intercourse*		
Agree	30.6	69.4
Disagree[†]	49.8	50.2
Don't Know	25.6	74.4
Most likely to get pregnant in first few days after period*		
Agree	42.7	57.3
Disagree[†]	53.1	46.9
Don't know	42.4	57.6
Cannot get pregnant going through change of life*		
Agree	57.6	42.4
Disagree[†]	47.0	53.0
Don't know	59.1	40.9

* $p < 0.001$.
†   Most appropriate response.

A logistic regression model was fitted for the discrete variable whether or not sex education was received. While the model did not provide a good fit, age, education, maternal status and social class were all found to be significant. These results support those found in the bivariate analysis — namely, that the likelihood of having received sex education is negatively associated with age and positively associated with social class.

Risk Factors Associated with the AIDS Virus

The issues addressed here are concerned with identifying *who* women consider to be particularly at risk of being infected with the AIDS virus and *what* approaches women consider to be most effective for sexually-active people to reduce the risk of being infected by the AIDS virus. In addressing these questions, survey respondents were asked to identify population groups that they considered to be at risk of being infected by the AIDS virus and also to specify how sexually-active people could reduce their risk of exposure to this virus.[1] The results presented in Table 3.7 show that 70 per cent and 60 per cent, respectively, of women consider that those injecting drugs and those who have casual sex/several partners are at risk of contracting the AIDS virus. In addition, one in every two women considers that homosexuals/bisexuals are at high risk for this virus. Less than 20 per cent of women identified the following individuals as being in the high-risk category: people having sexual intercourse with AIDS-infected people, unborn children of an infected woman, haemophiliacs, blood transfusion recipients and prostitutes. It is cause for concern that the proportion of women who said that they did not know what population groups were at risk for the AIDS virus is significantly related to age, education, employment status and medical-card

Table 3.7: Proportion of Women Identifying Specified Risk Groups for the AIDS Virus

Risk Groups for the AIDS Virus	*Proportion* %
Drug Abusers	70.2
Homosexuals/Bisexuals	53.4
Having Casual Sex/Several Partners	59.7
Sexual intercourse with partner infected with AIDS	19.7
Unborn children of infected woman	5.5
Haemophiliacs	16.9
Those receiving blood transfusions	13.1
Prostitutes	13.4
Other	10.7
Don't know	3.1

[1] Respondents could provide more than one answer to these questions on "risk factors for HIV infection" and "at risk groups" addressed in Section 3 of the questionnaire. All responses were noted, giving an average of 2.7 responses for the question on population groups considered most "at risk" of being infected with the AIDS virus and an average of 1.9 responses to the question on "risk minimising behaviour".

status. Over 3 per cent of women aged 25–29 and over the age of 40 do not know who is at risk of being infected with the AIDS virus. The proportion of women in this category declines from a high of 8 per cent for those with primary education to less than 1 per cent for women with third-level qualifications. The 6 per cent of women with medical cards who do not know who is at greatest risk of the AIDS virus drops to 2 per cent for women without medical cards. At 4.4 per cent, women on home duties account for the highest proportion in this category, by employment status.

Table 3.8 shows that the use of a condom is the most frequently specified approach for sexually-active people to reduce the risk of AIDS. While the use of condoms is specified by 82 per cent of women, only 43 per cent identified that staying with one partner was important in reducing the risk of AIDS. Avoidance of casual sex was specified by just 25 per cent, and other common approaches identified by between 7 and 16 per cent of women included: reducing the number of partners, abstaining from sexual intercourse and using safe sex practices. The proportion of women who did not know how to reduce the risk of AIDS was significantly related to age, educational level and medical-card status. Between 3 and 7 per cent of women aged between 40 and 60 could not identify approaches considered important for sexually-active people to reduce the risk of AIDS. A high of 8 per cent of women with primary education only and 6 per cent of medical-card holders were in a similar position. The fact that substantial numbers

Table 3.8: Proportion of Women Specifying Most Effective Approaches for Sexually-Active People to Reduce the Risk of Infection with the AIDS Virus

Approaches to Reduce the Risk of AIDS	Proportion (%)
Stay with one partner	42.8
Reduce number of partners	9.5
Use a condom	81.5
Abstain from sexual intercourse	15.3
Avoid casual sex	25.1
Use safe sex practices	7.4
Other	7.4
Don't know	2.8

of women still do not know what population groups are most at risk of the AIDS virus and how sexually-active people may reduce their risk of exposure to this virus is cause for serious concern and should be directly addressed by public health strategies aimed at reducing the incidence and the spread of this condition.

Conclusion

The finding that relatively more younger women than older women have received formal sex education is not surprising given the relatively recent introduction of sex education into the formal education system. What is, however, surprising and worrying is the fact that a substantial proportion of the female population still do not have accurate information on when they are at greatest risk of pregnancy. This information would have to be considered elementary and should be considered essential for all women. In addition, the level of awareness of the population groups most at risk of the AIDS virus and the most effective means of avoiding exposure to AIDS by sexually-active people is less than adequate. The finding that these factors are significantly related to level of education, employment status and medical-card status raises questions about the effectiveness of the channels through which this information is supposed to be imparted.

The information gaps in evidence from the findings presented here should warrant specific attention in any programmes aimed at informing women about the functioning of their own reproductive system. In particular, it would seem essential to ensure that sex education programmes aimed at post-pubescent girls specifically address all issues arising with regard to the risk of becoming pregnant. Ensuring that all sexually-active women are fully informed about the risk factors associated with infection by the AIDS virus and how these risks can be avoided must now be recognised as a public health priority. Given the finding that the knowledge gaps on this question vary according to level of education, employment status and medical-card status, there may be good grounds for targeting information programmes to those population groups where current levels of information are considered least adequate.

4

Family Planning

Introduction

The enactment of the Health (Family Planning) Act, 1979 removed
the ban on the sale of contraceptives in Ireland. While this ban was
in place prior to the passing of this legislation, nevertheless a high
proportion of married couples are reported to have practised some
form of "family limitation" (Wilson-Davis, 1975). Between the
passing of the 1979 legislation and the enactment of the most recent Health (Family Planning) (Amendment) Act, 1993, there has
been an increasing liberalisation of the conditions governing the
sale of contraceptives in this country. Under the most recent legislation, condoms can be sold in a wide variety of outlets and have
been removed from the scope of legislation that controls the availability of medical contraceptives. In the survey of women's health
needs in Ireland, the section on family planning addressed the
question of sexual activity, whether or not some form of family
planning was used and, if so, what method. In addition, questions
were asked about attitudes to the availability of contraceptives
and sterilisation services.

On the basis of the results forthcoming from this survey, two
out of every three women are sexually active. When analysed by
marital status, 90 per cent of married women are sexually active
compared with 26 per cent of single women and 18 per cent of
women who are separated, divorced or widowed. While 31 per cent
of women who are sexually active do not currently use any form of
family planning, this varies by marital status. One-third of
sexually-active married women do not use any family planning
compared with approximately one in every ten sexually-active
single women.

One in every two women thinks that family planning advice is accessible in her area, with over 80 per cent believing the information available to them to be adequate. The general practitioner (GP) was the source of choice for information on family planning by 44 per cent of women, while the family planning clinic was estimated to be the centre of choice for over a quarter of the female population. Close to one-third of women think that family planning advice should be available from their GP, with an additional 25 per cent citing the health centre and 22 per cent specifying the family planning clinic.

The most frequently used methods of family planning are condoms (22 per cent), followed by the combined pill (17 per cent), with the natural method in third place (14 per cent). The most frequently reported reason for changing the method of family planning used was the fear of side effects (30 per cent). Over 84 per cent of women think that condoms should be sold in Ireland without a prescription and, of these, 99 per cent think that they should be available in chemists, and between a half and two-thirds think that they should be available in a range of retail outlets. An estimated 82 per cent of women think that sterilisation should be available for both women and men in all publicly funded hospitals.

Access to Information on Family Planning

Following bivariate analyses, perceived accessibility to advice on family planning was found to vary significantly by age, employment status and geographical location. Medical-card status, social class and level of education achieved were found not to be significantly related to accessibility of family planning advice. The accessibility of family planning advice analysed by age group and employment status is shown in Table 4.1. With the exception of those aged 45–49 and 55–60, over one in every two women in all other age groups consider that family planning advice is accessible. Between one-quarter and one-third of women across the age groups are estimated to consider that family planning advice is not accessible. At 61 per cent, the highest proportion of women estimated to consider family planning advice accessible is found among those working part-time. Close to one-third of women who are unemployed believe that family planning advice is not accessible in their area. It is disturbing to note that when this question was asked of sexually-active women, one-third consider that advice on family planning was not easily accessible in their area.

Table 4.1: Accessibility of Family Planning Advice and Adequacy of Family Planning Information, by Age Group and Employment Status

	Accessibility of Family Planning Advice			Adequacy of Family Planning Information			
	Accessible	Not Accessible	Don't Know	Completely Adequate	Adequate	Inadequate	Very Inadequate
Age Group*	%	%	%	%	%	%	%
18–24	51.3	25.7	23.1	20.2	62.1	14.4	3.3
25–29	50.3	33.7	16.0	27.3	57.3	10.7	4.7
30–34	55.3	32.0	12.7	24.4	55.8	14.7	5.2
35–39	56.1	27.5	16.4	29.0	52.2	14.6	4.3
40–44	53.0	31.9	15.1	23.5	56.5	13.4	6.6
45–49	44.7	35.5	19.9	20.2	58.8	15.5	5.5
50–54	50.5	24.0	25.4	17.9	64.0	12.1	6.0
55–60	39.4	23.0	37.5	17.5	68.7	10.4	3.4
All	50.6	29.2	20.2	22.9	59.1	13.4	4.7
*Employment Status** *							
Working Full-time	47.8	28.9	23.3	22.1	60.7	12.6	4.6
Working Part-time	60.5	26.6	12.8	25.2	59.8	11.6	3.4
Unemployed	48.9	31.3	19.8	23.2	52.2	19.0	5.7
Home Duties	51.6	29.9	18.5	24.2	58.5	12.4	5.0
Students/ Retired/Ill/ Disabled	49.9	27.3	22.9	16.3	59.5	20.3	4.0
All	50.6	29.2	20.2	22.9	59.1	13.4	4.7

*   Age Group by Accessibility of Family Planning Advice: $p < 0.001$.
    Age Group by Adequacy of Family Planning Information: $p < 0.005$.
** $p < 0.05$

Table 4.2 shows the accessibility of family planning advice analysed by Health-Board area and geographical location. It is estimated that over half the women in the Health Boards of the East, the Midland, the North West and the South consider that family planning advice is accessible in their areas. This contrasts with an estimate of around one-third for the North Eastern and South Eastern Health Boards. The proportion of women who consider that family planning advice is not accessible in their area ranges from 22 per cent in the Midland Health Board to 39 per cent in the South Eastern Health Board. A strong urban/rural contrast is also in evidence in Table 4.2 with over one-third of rural women believing that family planning advice is not accessible, compared with one-quarter of women living in urban areas.

Table 4.2: Accessibility of Family Planning Advice and Adequacy of Family Planning Information, by Health-Board Area and Urban/Rural Location

	Accessibility of Family Planning Advice			Adequacy of Family Planning Information			
	Accessible	Not Ac-cessible	Don't Know	Completely Adequate	Adequate	Inadequate	Very In-adequate
Health-Board Area*	%	%	%	%	%	%	%
East	55.4	24.0	20.6	26.9	55.4	12.2	5.6
Midland	55.6	21.8	22.6	37.0	48.5	12.0	2.4
Mid-West	47.1	35.3	17.6	21.7	60.3	14.1	3.9
North-East	33.8	35.5	30.6	12.8	63.7	18.8	4.7
North-West	54.4	25.0	20.6	13.1	69.5	13.2	4.1
South	54.8	31.4	13.8	18.1	69.0	9.2	4.5
South-East	38.9	39.2	21.9	30.6	51.5	13.5	4.4
West	47.2	34.3	18.5	18.8	57.1	19.4	4.6
All	50.6	29.2	20.2	22.9	59.1	13.4	4.7
Geographical Location*							
Rural	42.0	37.7	20.4	18.3	62.2	14.4	5.1
Urban	56.1	23.8	20.1	25.8	57.1	12.7	4.5
All	50.6	29.2	20.2	22.9	59.1	13.4	4.7

* p < 0.001.

Tables 4.1 and 4.2 show that the perceived adequacy of the family planning advice available also varied significantly by age, employment status, and Health-Board area. Medical-card status, education level and social class were found not to have a significant relationship to this variable. In total, around 80 per cent of the women across all age groups find the family planning advice available to be completely adequate or adequate. The proportion of women estimated to consider the family planning advice to be inadequate increases as age rises to 50. The perceived adequacy of family planning information is reported to be highest for women who are working/engaged in home duties, and lowest for unemployed women, students, the retired, and those who are ill/ disabled.

Table 4.2 shows that just over three-quarters of the women in the North Eastern and Western Health Boards think that the available family planning information is completely adequate or adequate. For the other health-board areas, in excess of 80 per cent of women are found within these categories. The 14 per cent of women in the Midland Health-Board area who think that the family planning information is inadequate contrasts with the findings of a 1995 study of women of child-bearing age in this region. In the survey conducted for the Midland Health Board, 39 per cent of women said that the family planning services in the area were either poor or very poor (Midland Health Board). The fact that the Midland Health-Board study was specifically concerned with the provision of family planning services by GPs in the area may have had a bearing on the results. At 83 per cent, the proportion of urban women who consider the family planning advice to be adequate is slightly higher than that for rural women.

The source of information on family planning was found to vary significantly by age, medical-card status, level of education, employment status, geographical location and social class. The estimates presented in Table 4.3 indicate that the GP, followed by the family planning clinic, would be most frequently used for information on family planning. While the GP would be consulted by an estimated 36 per cent of those aged 18–24, the proportion is in the region of 44–49 per cent for those aged 25–45. One in every four women would use the family planning clinic as the source of family planning information. It is interesting to note that between 5 and 10 per cent of women aged under 50 would not seek family planning information locally. When the variation by medical-card status is reviewed in Table 4.3, it is interesting that it is in the use of the health centre and local information that the main differences occur. While 13 per cent of medical-card holders specify the health centre as the source of family planning information, this contrasts with the 9 per cent estimated for non-medical-card holders. Just less than 11 per cent of non-medical-card holders would not seek information locally, compared with an estimated 8 per cent of medical-card holders.

The analysis by level of education and employment status presented in Table 4.4 again shows that the GP and the family planning clinic would be most frequently consulted for information

Table 4.3: Where Information on Family Planning Would Be Obtained, by Age Group, and Medical-Card Status

Source of Information on Family Planning	Age Group*									Medical-Card Status*		
	18–24	25–29	30–34	35–39	40–44	45–49	50–54	55–60	All	Yes	No	All
	%	%	%	%	%	%	%	%	%	%	%	%
GP	36.2	46.4	46.4	48.3	44.4	42.1	45.2	44.1	43.6	43.7	43.5	43.5
Hospital	1.7	2.5	2.2	1.5	2.6	2.6	3.1	1.4	2.2	2.5	2.1	2.2
Health Centre	10.1	8.6	9.6	10.9	9.4	11.9	13.1	9.3	10.2	13.3	9.0	10.3
Family Planning Clinic	27.3	28.7	27.0	24.8	27.8	24.9	20.1	19.3	25.7	23.4	26.3	25.4
Public Health Nurse	0.4	1.4	1.4	2.0	1.5	1.3	0.3	1.2	1.2	1.8	1.0	1.2
Pharmacy	0.8	0.2	1.2	1.1	1.1	0.5	0.3	0.3	0.8	0.5	0.9	0.7
Family	6.6	1.1	1.2	0.7	0.4	1.2	0.0	0.5	2.0	1.7	2.1	2.0
Other	5.7	4.6	3.9	4.4	3.2	4.6	4.2	4.8	4.5	5.1	4.2	4.4
Would not seek information locally	10.8	6.6	6.9	5.7	8.8	10.4	12.4	18.9	9.6	7.6	10.7	9.8
Information not available locally	0.3	0.0	0.2	0.5	0.8	0.5	1.2	0.2	0.4	0.6	0.3	0.4

* $p < 0.001$.

on family planning. At 34 per cent, the use of the GP by the "other" employment status group, which includes students, the retired, the ill/disabled and others not in the labour force, is substantially lower than the estimates for all other categories. The use of the family planning clinic is highest for those working part-time. The use of the health centre is again lowest for the "other" employment status category, with an estimate of 6 per cent, compared with 12 per cent for the unemployed and those on home duties. The fact that it is the "other" category that is estimated to have the highest proportion (16 per cent) who would not seek

Table 4.4: Source of Family Planning Information, by Education Level and Employment Status

	Source of Family Planning Information							
	GP	Hospital	Health Centre	Family Planning Clinic	Public Health Nurse	Pharmacy	Other	Would not seek locally
Education Level*	%	%	%	%	%	%	%	%
Primary Cert/Lower	41.8	2.5	12.4	25.9	1.6	0.2	5.5	10.1
Inter/Group/ Junior Cert	44.3	2.9	13.2	23.3	1.2	0.9	5.3	9.0
Leaving Cert/ Matric	43.0	1.9	8.6	26.2	1.2	1.1	8.4	9.6
Qualification from RTC, etc.	45.6	0.9	7.3	27.8	0.4	0.2	7.9	9.9
University Qualification	46.4	1.1	4.6	29.4	0.4	0.4	7.8	10.0
All	43.5	2.2	10.2	25.7	1.2	0.7	6.9	9.6
*Employment Status**								
Working Full-time	44.0	1.8	8.6	26.8	0.9	1.0	7.1	9.9
Working Part-time	43.5	1.0	10.4	30.6	1.6	1.0	5.1	6.9
Unemployed	40.3	2.3	11.5	27.1	0.0	0.6	8.4	9.7
Home Duties	45.4	2.7	12.0	23.5	1.7	0.6	5.5	8.6
Students/Retired/ Ill/Disabled	34.2	1.5	6.0	28.1	0.2	0.7	13.8	15.6
All	43.6	2.2	10.2	25.7	1.2	0.8	7.1	9.6

* p < 0.001.

information locally is consistent with the general trend in evidence for this group. The data available for the source of information on family planning by educational experience show that as the level of education increases, the use of the health centre is likely to decrease. There is very little difference by educational level in terms of the willingness to seek information locally.

From Table 4.5 there is some geographical variation in evidence in the source of information on family planning. The estimates for the proportion who would consult the GP varies from a low of 39 per cent in the Mid-West to a high of 55 per cent in the Midland Health Board. The use of the family planning clinic also seems to vary by health-board area, though geographical variations in the availability of this service must also be recognised. It is estimated that just 9 per cent of women in the North East would use the family planning clinic for information, compared with a high of 39 per cent in the Mid-West. The GP and the family planning clinic would seem to be operating as alternative options at the health-board level. It is of some concern to note from Table 4.5 that 23 per cent of women in the North East would not seek information on family planning locally. The fact that the GP is the source of family planning information for more rural women and the family planning clinic is used by more urban women may be influenced as much by availability as by choice between these facilities.

The variation in the centre of choice for family planning information by social class shown in Table 4.5 is particularly interesting for the health centre option. This option is clearly more likely to be the preferred choice for women from the manual groups compared with those from the non-manual groups. Between 20 and 30 per cent of women across all social classes would attend the family planning clinic for family planning information.

Some interesting findings emerged from an analysis of source of family planning information by marital status, and whether or not the women had ever had a baby. Single women are more likely to use the family planning clinic, while married women are more likely to go to the GP. Just over one-fifth of sexually-active single women not currently using family planning have had a baby, compared with 86 per cent of married women. While 47 per cent of all mothers specified the GP as the source of family planning information, this contrasted with the estimate of 38 per cent for women who had not had a baby. Over 13 per cent of the latter

Table 4.5: Source of Family Planning Information, by Health-Board Area, Urban/Rural Location and Social Class

	Source of Family Planning Information							
	GP	*Hospital*	*Health Centre*	*Family Planning Clinic*	*Public Health Nurse*	*Pharmacy*	*Other*	*Would not seek locally*
*Health-Board Area**	%	%	%	%	%	%	%	%
East	41.8	2.4	7.7	29.1	0.5	1.0	7.9	9.7
Midland	54.6	5.6	19.7	12.1	1.7	0.0	5.4	0.9
Mid-West	39.4	1.0	5.3	38.7	2.8	0.3	4.2	7.6
North-East	45.4	3.8	11.0	9.1	1.9	1.1	4.8	23.0
North-West	50.2	1.4	14.4	19.2	2.3	0.3	7.3	4.9
South	40.5	1.3	8.3	30.9	0.9	0.8	7.5	2.1
South-East	52.1	2.3	16.5	14.3	2.2	0.5	3.5	1.3
West	42.6	1.0	14.9	24.6	1.1	0.5	8.0	7.4
All	43.6	2.2	10.2	25.7	1.2	0.8	7.1	9.6
*Geographical Location**								
Rural	46.7	2.2	12.7	19.9	2.1	0.6	7.1	9.9
Urban	41.9	2.1	8.9	28.7	0.7	0.8	7.5	9.4
All	43.6	2.2	10.2	25.7	1.2	0.8	7.1	9.6
*Social Class**								
Higher Professional	47.1	2.6	7.0	27.7	1.1	0.7	4.1	9.1
Lower Professional	45.1	1.6	6.7	28.1	1.1	0.9	6.8	9.7
Other Non-Manual	43.5	2.6	8.8	26.8	1.5	1.0	6.5	9.3
Skilled Manual	46.9	1.8	16.9	23.6	0.9	0.7	4.0	5.2
Semi-Skilled Manual	41.6	2.4	12.6	24.8	1.3	0.4	8.2	8.7
Unskilled Manual	46.6	1.8	13.3	20.4	1.4	0.4	6.6	9.5
All	44.4	2.2	10.3	25.9	1.3	0.7	6.4	8.7

* $p < 0.001$.

group also reported that they would not seek this information locally, compared with 8 per cent for mothers.

The perceived adequacy of the family planning information received was estimated for each source and is presented in Table 4.6. For the six centres reviewed here, the lowest level of perceived adequacy — 70 per cent — was estimated for the pharmacy as a source of family planning information. It should be noted from Table 4.3, however, that just a very small proportion of women depend on the pharmacy for this information. For the other centres, in excess of 85 per cent of women are estimated to consider that the family planning information received is adequate.

Table 4.6: Adequacy of Family Planning Information Received, by Source of Information

Source of Family Planning Information*	Adequacy of Family Planning Information Received			
	Completely Adequate	Adequate	Inadequate	Very Inadequate
	%	%	%	%
GP	25.6	59.7	11.6	3.2
Hospital	20.4	69.7	8.7	1.2
Health Centre	19.5	68.7	10.0	1.8
Family Planning Clinic	27.6	62.5	6.9	3.0
Public Health Nurse	29.0	60.9	10.2	0.0
Pharmacy	21.0	49.0	12.9	17.2
Other	13.4	64.7	14.6	7.2
Would not seek locally	4.8	53.1	28.8	13.4
All	22.9	59.1	13.4	4.7

* p < 0.001.

Views on where family planning advice should be made available varied significantly by age, medical-card status, level of education, employment status and geographical location. Table 4.7 shows that the GP, the health centre and the family planning clinics are the centres which the majority of women believe should be providing family planning advice. While the GP ranks highest across all age groups, the family planning clinic is the second choice for the under 30s, with the health centre occupying second place for those aged over 30. It is interesting that more younger women believe that family planning information should be available in schools, though the estimates decline with increasing age groups. Table 4.7 shows that the GP is also the first preference for family planning information, irrespective of medical-card status. The health centre, however, receives higher preference from medical-card holders, while the family planning clinic ranks slightly higher for non-medical-card holders.

Table 4.7: Where Family Planning Advice Should Be Available, by Age Group and Medical-Card Status

	Where Family Planning Advice Should Be Available					
	GP	*Hospital*	*Health Centre*	*Well-Woman Clinic/Family Planning Clinic*	*Public Health Nurse*	*Other*
Age Group*	*%*	*%*	*%*	*%*	*%*	*%*
18–24	29.0	9.2	20.6	25.5	3.2	5.5
25–29	30.7	8.7	24.6	24.9	3.1	5.1
30–34	32.7	9.4	24.8	20.0	4.1	4.5
35–39	32.4	7.8	29.1	19.4	3.7	3.1
40–44	31.6	7.9	26.8	23.0	4.3	2.6
45–49	29.7	8.5	27.9	21.5	5.5	3.1
50–54	33.0	6.7	29.1	20.0	3.6	5.5
55–60	34.2	12.1	23.4	19.7	4.7	2.9
All	31.4	8.8	25.3	22.2	3.9	8.3
Medical-Card Status*						
Yes	31.1	9.4	27.5	19.0	5.3	3.7
No	31.6	8.5	24.7	23.4	3.4	4.1
All	31.5	8.7	25.5	22.1	3.9	8.3

*   p < 0.001

Table 4.8 shows that, irrespective of level of education, over 30 per cent of women consider that family planning information should

be available from the GP. As level of education increases, the preference for the health centre drops from 26 per cent to 24 per cent,
while the preference for the family planning centre peaks at 25 per
cent for the group with an RTC-level qualification. The suggestion
that family planning information should be available in schools receives highest support from those with university qualifications.
For the first four categories of employment status shown in Table
4.8, the GP, the health centre and the family planning clinic are
ranked in that order in terms of the support estimated for them as
sources of family planning information. For the "other" category of
employment status, including students, the retired and the

**Table 4.8: Where Family Planning Advice Should Be
Available, by Education Level and Employment Status**

	Where Family Planning Advice Should Be Available					
	GP	*Hospital*	*Health Centre*	*Well Woman Clinic / Family Planning Clinic*	*Public Health Nurse*	*Other*
Education Level*	%	%	%	%	%	%
Primary Cert/Lower	31.6	10.1	26.1	21.6	3.8	6.8
Inter/Group/Junior Cert	32.5	8.2	28.4	20.5	3.8	6.6
Leaving Cert/Matric	30.5	9.2	23.6	23.1	4.1	9.6
Qualification from RTC, etc.	30.9	5.8	22.9	25.4	3.0	11.9
University Qualification	30.5	7.9	23.9	22.6	4.0	11.0
All	31.3	8.8	25.3	22.2	3.9	8.5
Employment Status*						
Working Full-time	32.1	8.4	24.3	23.4	3.4	8.5
Working Part-time	29.8	8.5	25.7	23.2	2.8	10.1
Unemployed	29.5	10.9	26.8	19.8	1.6	11.5
Home Duties	32.0	9.2	26.9	20.7	4.6	6.7
Students/Retired/Ill/ Disabled	27.4	7.9	18.9	25.6	4.5	15.8
All	31.4	8.8	25.3	22.2	3.9	8.3

* $p < 0.001$.

ill/disabled, the family planning clinic received a high estimate of 26 per cent, with the health centre receiving a low estimate of 19 per cent. At 9 per cent, this group also provides the strongest support for the school as a source of information in this area.

The estimated preference for the source of family planning information by geographical location is presented in Table 4.9. While the GP is again among the most popular sources of such information, the fact that an estimated 35 per cent of women would use the health centre in the Midland Health Board is something of a deviation from the general trend. The preference for the health centre also reaches the 30 per cent level in the North Eastern and the South Eastern Health Boards. This trend contrasts with the relatively low ranking of the family planning clinic in these areas, though the geographical variations in the availability of this service must again be taken into account. Around 7 per cent of the women in the Midland and the Southern Health Boards consider that family planning information should also be available from the schools. The urban/rural variation is again most marked with the support for the health centres and the family planning clinics. While support for the health centre is strongest among rural women, the family planning clinics receive relatively more support from women based in urban areas. Proximity, in addition to preference, may, however, have a bearing on the differences observed for urban and rural women.

The independent variables found to be significant in the bivariate analyses were incorporated into a multivariate model estimated on whether or not respondents considered the family planning advice in the area to be easily accessible or not. As the dependent variable is discrete, a logistic regression model was fitted. Parameter estimates for the model are given in Table A4 in Appendix 3. The model does not provide a good fit, though there are some interesting results worthy of comment. While half the women in the country consider family planning advice to be easily accessible in their area, 20 per cent of women are unaware of the services available to them. The number of those who are unfamiliar with the locally available services increases as age increases. It is among women working full-time that the poorest level of awareness is evident. Part-time working women are the group most familiar with local services. This group also contains the highest proportion who consider advice to be easily accessible. A higher proportion of women living in urban areas consider family planning advice to be easily accessible than is the case among their rural counterparts. The North West is the Health Board with the highest proportion of women who consider family planning advice to be easily accessible, with the South East being the Health-Board area with the highest proportion of women who consider family planning advice not to be easily accessible. The North Eastern Health Board contains the highest proportion of women who are unaware of what is available to them locally.

Table 4.9: Where Family Planning Advice Should Be Available, by Health-Board Area and Geographical Location

	Where Family Planning Advice Should Be Available					
	GP	Hospital	Health Centre	Well Woman Clinic/Family Planning Clinic	Public Health Nurse	Other
Health-Board Area*	%	%	%	%	%	%
East	30.5	10.3	23.0	25.6	3.1	7.6
Midland	30.9	7.3	35.5	16.9	4.6	4.8
Mid-West	37.0	5.7	22.3	21.3	3.4	10.3
North-East	34.4	11.2	29.5	15.1	4.1	5.8
North-West	27.2	7.7	27.4	26.4	5.3	6.1
South	31.5	6.5	21.7	24.6	3.2	12.6
South-East	35.7	5.8	32.3	15.4	3.6	7.3
West	28.7	9.5	27.4	15.2	7.6	11.8
All	31.4	8.8	25.3	22.2	3.9	8.3
Geographical Location*						
Rural	32.0	7.8	29.7	17.7	5.2	7.5
Urban	31.0	9.4	22.9	24.5	3.2	9.0
All	31.4	8.8	25.3	22.2	3.9	8.3

* $p < 0.001$.

While there are other unmeasured variables having an effect on the perception of the accessibility of family planning services, some examples of predicted probabilities emerging from this multivariate model are presented in Table 4.10. The information in this table is intended to illustrate the strong effect that variables like geographical location have on the probability of the response. Table 4.10 shows that while 41 per cent of women working full-time, aged between 25 and 29 years and living in an urban area in the South Eastern Health Board would be expected to respond positively to the question on the accessibility of family planning advice, for another group of women of the same age and living in a rural area in the same health board, just 25 per cent would be expected

Table 4.10: Do Women Think that Family Planning is Accessible Locally? Estimated Percentages for Women with Selected Characteristics Defined According to Age, Work Force Participation, Geographical and Health-Board Area of Residence

	Women with Specified Characteristics	*Do You Think that Family Planning Advice is Easily Accessible in Your Area?*	
		Yes %	*No* %
1.	Age 25–29 Full-time Urban Area South Eastern H.B.	41	39
2.	Age 25–29 Full-time Rural Area South Eastern H.B.	25	58
3.	Age 25–29 Full-time Rural Area North Western H.B.	48	34
4.	Age 25–29 Part-time Rural Area North Western H.B.	57	34
5.	Age 55–60 Part-time Rural Area North Western H.B.	49	21

to respond positively. The next section will consider the methods
of family planning most frequently used by Irish women given access to this service.

Methods of Family Planning Used

An estimated one-third of women avail of family planning advice.
This varies significantly with age and ranges from about 20 per
cent in the 18–24 group to a high of around a half in the 25–35
group. In bivariate analysis, the method of family planning used
by sexually-active women was shown to vary significantly by age,
marital status, level of education, employment status, geographical location and social class. The association between age and the
method of family planning used is clearly demonstrated in Table
4.11 where the use of the natural method increases from an estimated low of 1.3 per cent among the 18–24 year olds, to a high of
25 per cent among women aged 45–49. The use of the combined
pill and condoms is highest for the younger age groups, with utilisation of these methods declining with increasing age. Given an
estimate of 45 per cent, the use of the combined pill is highest
among the 18–24 year olds, with utilisation declining sharply
among those aged 35 and over. While 31 per cent of the 18–24
group report the use of condoms, utilisation of this method ranges
between an estimate of one-quarter and one-fifth for those aged
between 25 and 50. Sterilisation is understandably rare among
the younger women, and reaches a peak at an estimated 13 per
cent for women in the 40–44 age group. The age factor is clearly in
evidence where it is reported that no method of family planning is
used. Sexually-active women who do not use family planning account for a steadily increasing proportion of each age group,
ranging from 12 per cent of the 18–24 group, to 26 per cent of the
35–39 group and 38 per cent of those aged between 45 and 49.

It is clear from Table 4.11 that there are significant differences
in the methods of family planning used by single women and
married women. While 39 per cent of single women opt for the
combined pill, the estimate for married women is just 12 per cent.
Close to one-third of single women use condoms, compared with
one-fifth of married women. The use of the natural approach is
almost non-existent among single women, while three times as
many married women as single women do not use any method of
family planning. Medical-card status was not a significant factor
in the method of family planning used.

Table 4.11: Method of Family Planning Used by the Sexually Active, by Age Group and Marital Status†

| | Age Group* | | | | | | | | Marital Status* | | |
	18–24	25–29	30–34	35–39	40–44	45–49	50–60	All	Single	Ever Married	All
	%	%	%	%	%	%	%	%	%	%	%
Natural	1.3	5.4	12.8	15.4	17.2	24.8	18.4	14.1	1.5	17.4	14.1
Coil/IUD	0.0	2.3	1.5	2.3	3.8	3.2	1.6	2.2	0.0	2.7	2.2
Diaphragm	0.6	0.2	0.7	1.9	1.9	0.5	0.3	0.9	0.0	1.1	0.9
Withdrawal	0.0	1.1	0.9	1.0	2.5	3.3	1.0	1.4	0.0	1.7	1.4
Combined Pill	44.8	35.2	24.6	11.6	5.2	3.4	0.9	16.6	39.4	11.9	16.6
Mini Pill	9.8	10.0	8.8	5.4	2.4	1.4	0.7	5.4	16.9	4.1	5.4
Condom	30.6	26.2	26.4	26.8	22.5	20.2	5.7	22.4	31.1	21.1	22.4
Sterilisation	1.0	3.7	3.3	9.6	13.3	5.7	2.5	5.9	0.9	7.5	5.9
None	12.0	16.0	20.9	26.0	30.5	37.6	68.8	30.9	10.2	32.4	30.9

* p < 0.001.

† Analysis based on 2,001 (67.2 per cent) women in the sample who are sexually active.

In reviewing the results by level of education in Table 4.12, it is clear that the use of the combined pill peaks at 21 per cent for those with RTC-level qualifications. At an estimate of just less than 19 per cent, this method of family planning is also frequently used by women with leaving certificate or university qualifications. It is interesting that for women with primary certificate, the estimates for the use of the natural method or condoms are similar at 13 per cent and 15 per cent, respectively. The estimates for the use of condoms range between 23 per cent and 30 per cent for women with higher levels of education. The highest level of use of the natural method is estimated at 16 per cent and is found for those with leaving certificate or university qualifications. Of those women who say that they are sexually active, it is estimated that 43 per cent of women with a primary education only are not using any method of family planning, compared with 21 per cent of women with a university qualification.

Women and Health Care in Ireland

Table 4.12: Method of Family Planning Used, by Education Level and Employment Status[†]

	Method of Family Planning Used								
	Natu-ral	Coil / IUD	Dia-phragm	With-drawal	Com-bined Pill	Mini Pill	Con-dom	Steri-lisation	None
Education Level*	%	%	%	%	%	%	%	%	%
Primary Cert/ Lower	13.3	3.1	0.4	1.7	11.0	4.2	14.8	7.9	43.4
Inter/Group/ Junior Cert	12.9	3.0	1.0	1.8	17.4	4.3	22.7	6.5	30.4
Leaving Cert/Matric	16.0	1.5	1.1	1.1	18.1	7.2	24.5	4.3	26.2
Qualification for RTC, etc.	9.4	0.0	0.0	0.0	21.2	5.9	27.0	5.9	30.7
University Qualification	15.5	0.9	1.9	1.5	18.8	4.0	29.6	7.9	20.5
All	14.2	2.2	0.9	1.4	16.5	5.4	22.3	6.0	31.0
*Employment Status**									
Working Full-time	11.9	1.7	0.7	1.1	22.9	6.9	26.6	2.3	25.9
Working Part-time	14.1	3.1	1.7	1.1	14.0	7.6	19.9	10.3	27.8
Unemployed	0.0	0.0	0.0	0.0	28.1	15.2	30.1	3.4	23.2
Home Duties	16.4	2.6	1.1	1.8	12.1	3.9	19.3	7.6	35.1
Student/Retired/ Ill/Disabled	8.1	0.0	0.0	0.0	33.7	3.7	37.2	1.2	16.3
All	14.1	2.2	0.9	1.4	16.6	5.4	22.4	5.9	30.9

*   p < 0.001.

†   Analysis by education level limited to the 1,993 (67.4 per cent) women in the sample who are sexually active for whom education level attained is available.

Analysis by employment status limited to the 2,001 (67.2 per cent) women in the sample who are sexually active.

Table 4.12 shows that the "other" employment category accounts for the highest estimates of the use of the combined pill and condoms, at 34 per cent and 37 per cent respectively. More than one-quarter of unemployed women are estimated to use the combined pill, with 30 per cent of this group using condoms. Sterilisation is the option chosen by an estimated 10 per cent of women working part-time. Over one-third of women in the home duties category are not using any method of family planning, with 16 per cent of this group using the natural approach.

Geographical variation in the method of family planning of choice is shown in Table 4.13. There are some interesting patterns, with the use of the combined pill estimated at the highest level of around 20 per cent in the East and the Midlands and lowest, at approximately 13 per cent, in the Mid-West and the North West. The use of condoms varies between one-fifth and one-quarter, with the exception of the Midlands, the North East and the West where the level drops below 20 per cent. The highest estimates for sterilisation are found in the Midlands and the South, at 9 per cent and 10 per cent, respectively. The use of the natural method is most common in the North West, the South East and the West, where estimates in the range 18–20 per cent are recorded. The lowest estimate of 26 per cent for the proportion of women not using any method of family planning is found in the East and contrasts with the highest estimate of 44 per cent found for the North East. In this category, estimates of at least one-third of sexually-active women not using any method of family planning are found for five of the health boards. The differences in approach used by rural and urban women summarised in Table 4.13 consolidate the patterns in evidence at the health-board level. When women are compared according to area of residence, urban women are more likely to use the combined pill and condoms and rural women are more likely to use the natural method of family planning. While more than a quarter of sexually-active women in urban areas do not use any form of family planning, this contrasts with the estimate of 37 per cent for women living in rural areas.

Table 4.13 shows quite a strong social class effect both on the use of family planning and on the specific method used. While 26 per cent of sexually-active women in the higher professional group say that they do not currently use family planning, the estimate for the other groups is in excess of 30 per cent, with a high of 37 per cent estimated for women in the skilled manual group. The combined pill is the most preferred choice for women in the semi-skilled group, while condoms are the first choice for women in the other groups. A higher proportion of women in the lower professional group choose the natural method of family planning relative to women in other social class categories.

Table 4.13: Method of Family Planning Used, by Health-Board Area, Geographical Location and Social Class[†]

	Method of Family Planning Used								
	Natu-ral	Coil/IUD	Dia-phragm	With-drawal	Com-bined Pill	Mini Pill	Con-dom	Steri-lisation	None
Health-Board Area*	%	%	%	%	%	%	%	%	%
East	11.9	1.7	1.0	2.2	19.7	7.0	24.6	6.0	25.6
Midland	13.0	1.1	0.8	0.7	20.6	4.5	18.0	9.0	32.4
Mid-West	14.8	3.4	2.7	0.6	13.1	3.2	25.7	3.4	33.2
North-East	11.0	2.2	1.5	0.6	14.6	2.4	18.9	4.8	44.0
North-West	19.6	2.4	0.8	0.7	12.4	5.7	21.4	2.7	34.5
South	13.6	3.0	0.1	1.4	15.1	4.8	23.7	9.8	28.5
South-East	20.4	2.4	0.0	1.9	13.9	5.2	20.6	5.5	29.4
West	17.9	2.3	0.5	0.0	14.1	4.7	17.2	3.9	39.5
All	14.1	2.2	0.9	1.4	16.6	5.4	22.4	5.9	30.9
*Geographical Location**									
Rural	18.1	2.8	0.9	1.2	12.6	5.2	18.4	4.1	36.6
Urban	11.8	1.8	0.9	1.5	19.1	5.5	24.8	7.0	27.4
All	14.1	2.2	0.9	1.4	16.6	5.4	22.4	5. 9	30.9
*Social Class**									
Higher Professional	17.3	1.6	1.1	2.5	13.8	4.7	24.9	7.8	26.2
Lower Professional	19.3	1.6	1.3	0.9	8.7	4.7	26.0	7.5	30.3
Other Non-Manual	14.8	2.4	1.1	0.8	17.2	5.8	21.4	4.3	32.0
Skilled Manual	11.6	2.3	0.7	2.8	15.2	5.6	16.5	8.3	37.0
Semi-Skilled Manual	7.8	2.8	0.7	0.9	26.8	5.6	20.1	5.1	30.3
Unskilled Manual	13.8	3.6	0.0	2.8	16.5	8.6	20.6	3.8	30.2
All	14.4	2.3	0.9	1.4	16.1	5.4	21.8	6.1	31.4

* $p < 0.001$.

†   Analysis by Health Board and geographical location limited to the 2,001 (67.2 per cent) women in the sample who are sexually active.
Analysis by social class limited to the 1,944 (71.4 per cent) women in the sample who are sexually active for whom social class is known.

A multivariate analysis was undertaken on the dependent variable whether or not family planning is used. As this is a discrete variable a logistic regression model was fitted. The variables education, marital status and urban/rural area of residence were found to be confounded within the age variable. Age, health-board area of residence and number of children were all significant, though the model was not a good fit as a substantial level of variation was left unexplained. Parameter estimates for this model are presented in Table A5 in Appendix 3. As this model is intended to predict the probability that family planning will not be used, these results indicate that while the use of family planning is generally inversely related to age, it is positively related to the number of children born. The estimates also show that the probability of using family planning is highest in the Eastern Health Board and lowest in the North Eastern Health Board. Table 4.14 shows some examples of estimated probabilities of using

Table 4.14: Estimated Percentages of Women who Use/Don't Use Family Planning for Women with Selected Characteristics Defined According to Age, Health-Board Area of Residence and Number of Children Born

Women with Specified Characteristics	*No Family Planning*	*Family Planning Used*
	%	%
1. Age 25–29 1 child Eastern Health Board	13	87
2. Age 25–29 1 child South Eastern Health Board	17	83
3. Age 25–29 4 children Mid-Western Health Board	10	90
4. Age 40–44 1 child Mid-Western Health Board	43	57
5. Age 40–44 4 children South Eastern Health Board	30	70

family planning for women with different characteristics. While
87 per cent of women aged 25–29 living in the Eastern Health-
Board area with one child are likely to use family planning, this
drops to an estimate of 57 per cent for women aged 40–44, with
one child, living in the Mid-Western Health-Board area.

Sale of Condoms

When asked specifically about their opinions regarding the sale of
condoms in Ireland, over 80 per cent of women under the age of 50
believe that condoms should be sold without a prescription. For
women under 40, the support for this proposition is in excess of
the 90 per cent level. Support drops in the older age groups with
an estimate of 69 per cent for those aged 50–54 and 54 per cent
for 50–60 year olds. Table 4.15 shows that support for the sale of
condoms only with a prescription is low among the younger age

**Table 4.15: Should Condoms be Sold in Ireland?, by Age
Group and Medical-Card Status**

	Should Condoms Be Sold in Ireland?		
	Yes, without a prescription	Yes, only with a prescription	No, should not be sold at all
Age Group*	%	%	%
18–24	92.2	6.4	1.4
25–29	92.2	7.5	0.3
30–34	93.3	6.0	0.8
35–39	89.5	8.7	1.8
40–44	87.7	8.4	4.0
45–49	80.1	14.4	5.5
50–54	68.9	20.5	10.6
55–60	54.1	28.7	17.2
All	84.4	11.3	4.3
*Medical-Card Status**			
Yes	77.4	14.7	8.0
No	87.0	10.2	2.9
All	84.1	11.5	4.4

* $p < 0.001$.

groups and increases to a high of 29 per cent among those aged 55–60. The oldest age group also provides the strongest support for the proposition that condoms should not be sold at all, which contrasts with the estimates of less than 4 per cent found for those aged under 45. It is probably not surprising that the higher support for the sale of condoms without a prescription is found for non-medical-card holders, as shown in Table 4.15.

For all categories of employment status, support for the sale of condoms without a prescription exceeds 80 per cent, with the estimate rising to a high of 92 per cent among the unemployed. Women with leaving certificate or third-level qualifications also provide strong support for this approach, with an estimate of around 90 per cent, though this drops to 73 per cent for women with a primary education only. Over 95 per cent of single women support the sale of condoms without a prescription, compared with 83 per cent for married women. The variation by health-board area presented in Table 4.16 is probably well summarised

Table 4.16: Should Condoms be Sold in Ireland?, by Health-Board Area, and Geographical Location

Health-Board Area*	Should Condoms Be Sold in Ireland?		
	Yes, without a prescription	*Yes, only with a prescription*	*No, should not be sold at all*
	%	%	%
East	93.6	4.7	1.7
Midland	84.4	12.2	3.4
Mid-West	83.7	13.2	3.2
North-East	74.6	17.3	8.1
North-West	71.9	18.9	9.2
South	82.7	11.8	5.5
South-East	82.8	11.5	5.7
West	72.7	21.7	5.6
All	84.4	11.3	4.3
*Geographical Location**			
Rural	74.3	18.5	7.2
Urban	90.9	6.7	2.5
All	84.4	11.3	4.3

* $p < 0.001$.

in the urban/rural dichotomy. Support for the sale of condoms without a prescription ranges from between 70 and 75 per cent in the North East, the North West and the West to 94 per cent in the East. For women in rural areas, this support is consolidated at the 74 per cent level, which contrasts with the 91 per cent estimated for women in urban areas.

Irrespective of age, medical-card status, level of education, employment status or geographical location, in excess of 98 per cent of women who support the sale of condoms in Ireland are in favour of the sale of condoms in chemists. Support from this group for supermarkets, other retail store or pubs/discos as outlets for the sale of condoms was lower and more varied. While on average an estimate of close to 60 per cent supported the use of the supermarket or other retail stores as sales outlets, this varied by age group, employment status, marital status and geographical location. Younger, working women living in urban areas were more supportive of this proposition. The estimate of the support for pubs/discos was averaged at a higher level of around two-thirds, though the profile of stronger support among the younger, working urban women remained consistent.

Sterilisation

The final issue raised in this review of family planning practices was whether or not sterilisation should be available to women and men in all publicly-funded hospitals. An estimated 82 per cent of women support the availability of sterilisation for both men and women in publicly-funded hospitals. While this support was significantly associated with age, medical-card status, level of education, employment status, geographical location and social class, the support for these services being available to both women and men was similar in all cases. In excess of three out of four women under the age of 55 support the provision of sterilisation in public hospitals. A similar level of support was estimated for medical-card holders, with an increase to a level of 85 per cent for non-medical-card holders. Irrespective of educational experience or employment status, the support for publicly-available sterilisation was again estimated to be in excess of the 77 per cent level. Higher levels of support were estimated among women who were working or unemployed and who had a minimum of an intermediate certificate education. Variation in support for the public availability of sterilisation for both men and women ranged from a high of around 87 per cent for women in the higher professional class to a low of 72 per cent for the unskilled manual group.

On a geographical basis, the lowest levels of support for the provision of sterilisation in public hospitals were estimated for the North East, the North West, the West and the South East. In all of these health-board areas, support was estimated to be between 70 and 75 per cent, which compared with estimates of between 82 and 89 per cent in the other health-board areas. This variation is again well represented in the urban/rural dichotomy, with support for publicly-available sterilisation estimated at 74 per cent for women resident in rural areas, and 87 per cent for women in urban areas.

Conclusion

The findings in this chapter regarding the use of family planning services by Irish women support those available from other studies, which indicate that such choices result from a complex of social, economic and personal factors (Matteson and Hawkins, 1993; Skjeldestad, 1993). The majority support for the widespread availability of condoms and easier access to sterilisation services indicates a liberalisation of attitudes to the availability of contraceptives, compared with the early to mid-1970s (Wilson-Davis, 1975).

What is indicated in the results reported here is perceived differences in the accessibility of family planning services by women in different parts of the country and in different social circumstances. These differences have persisted despite commitments to improving access to information on, and services for, family planning proposed by the *Report of the Second Commission on the Status of Women* (1993) and actively pursued by the Department of Health (Department of Health, 1995a). In pursuing the implementation of this objective, the Department of Health issued guidelines on family planning policy to health boards in March 1995. These guidelines for health boards are summarised here as they may be seen to constitute an extensive and official statement of family planning policy (Department of Health, 1995b):

(1) Each health board should ensure that an equitable, accessible and comprehensive family planning service is provided in its area.

(2) The role of the GP in providing family planning services is recognised and this role will be developed and strengthened.

(3) A broadly-based programme, involving family planning clinics provided by the health board and/or other service-providers, will be developed to ensure that services are within easy reach and that choice of service-provider is available.

(4) The family planning service in each maternity hospital/unit will be evaluated to determine the extent to which current needs are being met.

(5) Sterilisation operations for family planning purposes are a matter for decision by the individuals concerned in conjunction with their consultants. Where sterilisation is not available at a particular hospital, the patient has the right to ask her consultant to refer her to a hospital where the procedure is available and the health board should make the appropriate arrangements.

(6) Health boards should ensure that vasectomy services are available.

(7) Arrangements for the dissemination of information on family planning should be made by health boards. Copies of family planning materials, including those available from the Health Promotion Unit of the Department of Health, should be made available to the public through sources such as GPs, non-governmental organisations, maternity hospitals/units, pharmacies and health-board services.

(8) Each health board should provide a leaflet which outlines the type and range of family planning services available in its area and details of service providers or contact phone numbers.

(9) The range of services to be provided free of charge under the G.M.S. is being extended to include spermicidal contraceptives and contraceptive devices.

(10) The family planning requirements of individuals in deprived and/or at-risk groups, and of those with special needs, will be established by health boards, in consultation with the groups involved and provided in a manner that is easily understood by the recipients.

(11) Health boards will ensure that the family planning needs of persons living in remote areas are adequately met.

(12) Health boards should devise appropriate arrangements to ensure a co-ordinated approach in the development and implementation of the services (within health boards or between health boards).

From the information presented here, it is clear that the objective of equal access for all to family planning services has yet to be achieved. If the implementation of these guidelines will facilitate the achievement of these objectives, their application should be actively pursued by all health boards and by the Department of Health.

5

Gynaecology

Introduction

The appropriate use of preventive health services by women may help to avoid unnecessary morbidity associated specifically with the reproductive system. While research is ongoing on the effectiveness of certain types of screening services, basic information is available on how relatively low-cost services may most effectively be used to maintain good health (Department of Health, 1995a). In this part of the study, women were asked about the gynaecological services they used most frequently and the extent to which health promotion initiatives like cervical smear testing and breast self-examination were undertaken. In addition, the level of prevailing information on the menopause as an important life-cycle event was addressed. The main focus here is an assessment of the information that women have available to them, and the initiatives taken towards the objective of maintaining good physical health.

From the survey, it is estimated that 30 per cent of women had attended a gynaecologist, with the majority of these attending to have a smear taken (22 per cent) or because of heavy periods (15 per cent). In addition, close to 10 per cent reported attending because of irregular bleeding, while 7 per cent had sexual problems. With an estimate of 45 per cent, the majority of women consider that a smear should be taken every year, though the recommended frequency of two or three years was specified by a total of 44 per cent. While 65 per cent of women are estimated ever to have had a cervical smear, this test had been undergone within the previous 12 months by 31 per cent, within the previous one or two years by 29 per cent and in excess of three years by 26 per cent. An estimated 9 per cent of women had ever had an abnormal smear, while 6 per cent reported that a family member had ever had an abnormal smear and 4.2 per cent had a close female relative with cancer of the cervix. Close to 62 per cent of women have suffered from pre-menstrual tension, though this varies from 56 per cent for women with primary education only to 68 per cent for those with third-level qualifications. Among women who have had pre-menstrual tension, 37 per cent just suffer the symptoms, while 21 per cent deal with it by taking pain killers.

While 61 per cent of women consider that they have adequate information on the menopause, close to 20 per cent either do not know or do not have enough information on this condition. With regard to the symptoms of the menopause, hot flushes are indicated by almost one-third of women, termination of periods by one-quarter and irritability in the case of 18 per cent. The general practitioner is the information source for over half the population, with 12 per cent using the media and 11 per cent the family planning clinic. Just 7 per cent of women have had hormone replacement therapy, with over half acknowledging that this treatment may be prescribed to relieve the symptoms of the menopause. Over half the population of women would consider taking hormone replacement therapy during the menopause.

Close to one in four women performs self-examination of breasts frequently, with over one-third performing this examination occasionally and 39 per cent never conducting this examination. Of those who do not perform self-examination of breasts, 57 per cent have no particular reason for not doing so, while 17 per cent are afraid of what they might find and 10 per cent do not know what to do. While 42 per cent of women know that the week following the period is the best time to conduct breast self-examination, the same proportion of women do not know the best time of the month for this examination. Approximately 13 per cent of women have had a close female relative with breast cancer. With regard to the women who should have a mammogram, those aged over 40 and those who have breast lumps are each thought to be in need of this service by over 20 per cent of women. Women who have had a close female relative with breast cancer are also considered a priority by 18 per cent. Over half the population of women would not mind whether the doctor performing a breast examination was male or female while 43 per cent express a preference for a female doctor.

Almost 73 per cent of women know that osteoporosis is a gradual thinning of the bones. Close to 53 per cent and 19 per cent, respectively, consider that middle-aged/older women and older people are most at risk of this condition. An estimated one-fifth of women claim that they do not know the causes of this condition, the groups most at risk or the means of avoidance. Over half the population of women correctly identify lack of calcium as a cause of osteoporosis and taking a diet high in calcium as one way of avoiding the condition.

One out of every four women has experienced unavoidable leakage of urine and one-third of these consider that this is currently a problem. More than half of these women have sought help for this problem, with two-thirds going to the general practitioner for assistance. Close to 57 per cent of women who did not seek help for the condition had learned to live with it, while 14 per cent had been too embarrassed to do so.

More in-depth analysis of the issues covered in this area will be presented in the sections that follow.

Uptake of Gynaecology Services

Having a smear taken is the most frequently cited reason for attending a gynaecologist or gynaecological clinic. While it is generally recommended that women should have a cervical (or pap) smear test every two or three years, only two out of every three women have ever had a smear test and uptake varies significantly by age, employment status, educational experience, geographical location and social class.[1] There is, however, no significant relationship with medical-card status.

In Table 5.1, the proportion of women having had a smear test increases noticeably by age, from a low of 21 per cent for the 18–24 age group to in excess of 80 per cent for those aged between 30 and 55 years. The analysis by education level presented in Table 5.2 shows that a higher proportion of women with primary or intermediate-level education have had a smear test compared with those with more educational qualifications. Table 5.2 also shows that around 82 per cent of women working part-time or engaged in home duties have had a smear test compared with 15 per cent of those in the employment status category including students, the retired and the ill/disabled.

---

[1]   The recommended frequency of having a cervical smear (or pap smear) test may vary for the individual woman according to age and other factors.

Table 5.1: Ever Had a Cervical Smear Test, by Age Group

| | Ever Had a Cervical Smear Test | |
| | Yes | No |
Age Group*	%	%
18–24	20.6	79.5
25–29	55.3	46.7
30–34	80.1	20.0
35–39	86.4	13.6
40–44	84.2	15.8
45–49	79.3	20.7
50–54	81.9	18.1
55–60	63.9	36.1
All	65.2	34.8

*   p < 0.001.

Table 5.2: Ever Had a Cervical Smear Test, by Education Level and Employment Status

| | Ever Had a Cervical Smear Test | |
| | Yes | No |
Education Level*	%	%
Primary Cert/Lower	71.2	28.9
Inter/Group/Junior Cert	71.5	28.5
Leaving Cert/Matric	59.2	40.8
Qualification from RTC, etc.	53.1	47.0
University Qualification	65.1	34.9
All	65.1	34.8
*Employment Status**		
Working Full-time	53.5	46.5
Working Part-time	81.3	18.7
Unemployed	44.7	55.3
Home Duties	82.2	17.8
Student/Retired/Ill/Disabled	15.2	84.8
All	65.2	34.8

*   p < 0.001.

From the geographical variation in the uptake of smear tests in evidence in Table 5.3, it is clear that just over half the women in the Southern Health-Board area have ever had a smear test, compared with 71 per cent in the East. As a group, 62 per cent of rural women reported having had a smear test, while the equivalent

Table 5.3: Ever Had a Cervical Smear Test, by Health-Board Area, Geographical Location and Social Class

	Ever Had a Cervical Smear Test	
	Yes	No
*Health-Board Area**	%	%
East	70.6	29.4
Midland	69.3	30.7
Mid-West	60.2	39.8
North-East	66.5	33.5
North-West	66.3	33.7
South	51.5	48.5
South-East	68.3	31.7
West	63.1	36.9
All	65.2	34.8
*Geographical Location***		
Rural	61.8	38.2
Urban	67.1	32.9
All	65.2	34.8
*Social Class**		
Higher Professional	89.0	11.0
Lower Professional	76.8	23.2
Other Non-Manual	67.5	32.5
Skilled Manual	76.4	23.6
Semi-skilled Manual	57.0	43.0
Unskilled Manual	52.4	47.7
All	69.5	30.5

* $p < 0.001$.
** $p < 0.005$.

for urban women was estimated at 67 per cent. Married women and women who have had a baby are more likely to have had a smear test. While just 24 per cent of single women have had a smear test, the estimate for married women is 84 per cent. The comparison for women with/without children yielded a similar range, with 85 per cent of mothers having had a smear test compared with 28 per cent for women who have not had a baby.

The knowledge that women have regarding the recommended frequency for having a smear test is significantly associated with age, medical-card status, employment status, educational experience, geographical location and social class. In Table 5.4 estimates by age group are presented for the question on the recommended frequency for having a smear test. The variation in perceived frequency by age is seen quite clearly with over half the women in the 18–24 age group indicating that a woman should have a smear test once a year, while close to 40 per cent of the women over 35 years share the same opinion. The actual experience for the younger age group would seem to reflect the perception regarding the correct timing for having a smear test. Reality diverges from theory to some extent for the older age groups where between one-quarter and one-third of women aged between 35 and 55 have had a smear test within the previous year.

Close to half the women aged between 30 and 55 consider that a smear test should be taken either every two years or every three years. For women up to age 40, this corresponds reasonably closely to actual practice, though the proportion of women having a smear test over these intervals begins to decline in the older age groups. It would seem to be cause for concern that an estimated 18 per cent of women in the 18–24 age group and over 10 per cent of women aged over 50 respond "don't know" to this question. The proportion of women who had a smear test more than three years previously increases with age from 12 per cent for those aged 25–29, to 34 per cent for the 45–49-year-olds.

The time elapsed since the last smear test was not found to be significantly associated with medical-card status. The frequency with which a woman should have a smear test was, however, found to be significantly associated with this variable and the estimates are also reported in Table 5.4. While 31 per cent of those with medical cards fall within the "every two years" category, the comparable proportion for the non-medical-card holders is 35 per cent. Medical-card holders are more likely to respond that they "don't know" the answer to this question, with 8 per cent of non-medical-card holders estimated to fall into this category.

Table 5.4: Perception Regarding How Frequently a Woman Should Have a Cervical Smear Test,[†] by Age Group, Medical-Card Status and Social Class

Age Group*	Once a Year %	Every Two Years %	Every Three Years %	Less Often %	Don't Know %
18–24	54.5	21.7	5.6	0.3	17.9
25–29	49.3	33.2	9.3	0.6	7.6
30–34	49.4	36.5	10.1	0.6	3.4
35–39	39.0	39.9	14.1	2.6	4.4
40–44	38.6	39.9	13.2	1.8	6.5
45–49	43.8	38.2	9.2	2.7	6.1
50–54	40.2	38.4	10.5	0.7	10.2
55–60	38.8	32.3	12.3	1.2	15.5
All	45.3	34.0	10.2	1.2	9.3
Medical-Card Status*					
Yes	46.1	30.5	9.1	1.5	12.8
No	44.9	35.4	10.9	1.1	7.7
All	45.2	34.0	10.3	1.2	9.2
Social Class*					
Higher Professional	33.6	43.7	16.2	2.2	4.3
Lower Professional	40.1	42.8	11.6	1.5	4.0
Other Non-manual	44.2	35.4	10.6	1.3	8.4
Skilled Manual	48.7	33.9	9.7	1.8	6.1
Semi-skilled Manual	55.6	27.2	7.7	1.0	8.5
Unskilled Manual	37.0	32.3	10.4	0.0	20.3
All	44.6	35.8	10.6	1.3	7.7

*   p < 0.001.
†   While it is generally recommended that women have a smear test every 2/3 years, the recommended frequency for the individual may vary according to age and other factors.

Table 5.4 shows a clear social-class effect for women's knowledge regarding the recommended frequency for having a smear test. One of the most worrying findings from this table is that one in every five women from the unskilled manual group does not know the answer to this question and only 42 per cent answer within the correct range. The higher professional class accounts for the highest proportion of women indicating correctly that a smear test should be taken every two years or every three years.

Irrespective of employment status or educational experience, the highest proportion of women consider that a woman should have a smear test every year. From the estimates presented in Table 5.5, however, this would not seem to be borne out by practice. For all categories of employment status, the proportion of women having a smear test in the previous year was less than the proportion who considered annual smear tests to be the best standard. This was also the case for educational experience with the proportion of women having had a smear test in the previous year increasing from 22 per cent for those with primary education to 39 per cent for women with third-level qualifications. The unemployed and the category including students, the retired and the ill/disabled were the only groups for which the estimate of having had a smear test in the previous two years exceeded that which was considered desirable. For all levels of educational experience, the estimates for those who had a smear test in the previous two years tended to be lower than what was perceived as desirable, while the opposite was true for the three-year time interval.

Table 5.5 shows however, that there is some variation for these variables in the level of knowledge about utilisation of this service. While 13 per cent of women with a primary education say that they "don't know" how often a woman should have a smear test, this drops to about 8 per cent for those with third-level education. This factor seems to be reflected in experience, with 38 per cent of women with primary education not having had a smear test within the previous three years. For employment status, the "don't know" response is estimated at similar levels for working and unemployed women, with the highest proportion of 24 per cent estimated for the group including students, the retired and the ill/disabled. This latter group is also shown to include the highest proportion (36 per cent) of women who have not had a smear test in the previous three years. The estimate of 13 per cent

Table 5.5: Frequency of Having a Cervical Smear Test and Length of Time since Last Smear Test, by Education Level, Employment Status and Geographical Location

	Frequency of Having a Cervical Smear Test					How Long since Last Cervical Smear Test?[†]			
	Once a year	Every 2 yrs	Every 3 yrs	Less often	Don't now	Less than 12 mths	1–2 yrs	2–3 yrs	More than 3 yrs
*Education Level**	%	%	%	%	%	%	%	%	%
Primary Cert/Lower	45.2	30.6	9.8	1.1	13.3	21.3	27.5	13.7	37.5
Inter/Group/ Junior Cert	46.4	34.4	10.8	0.7	7.8	32.1	26.3	16.8	24.8
Leaving Cert/Matric.	44.8	35.2	10.7	1.4	7.9	33.9	31.9	12.8	21.3
Qualification from RTC etc.	49.9	33.0	6.5	2.6	8.0	39.3	24.8	14.6	21.3
University Qualification	43.2	36.8	9.3	2.0	8.8	38.7	35.1	11.2	15.0
All	45.4	34.0	10.2	1.3	9.1	31.0	29.2	14.1	25.7
*Employment Status***									
Working Full-time	47.3	32.9	8.9	0.8	10.1	39.9	30.4	11.1	18.7
Working Part-time	44.7	37.0	12.6	2.5	3.2	30.1	28.2	14.9	26.8
Unemployed	50.2	26.5	9.0	2.8	11.6	24.7	41.2	10.3	23.8
Home Duties	41.5	38.4	12.0	1.4	6.7	27.8	28.2	15.8	28.2
Student/ Retired/Ill/ Disabled	56.2	15.3	4.2	0.7	23.7	16.5	29.3	17.7	36.5
All	45.3	34.0	10.2	1.2	9.2	31.0	29.2	14.3	25.5
*Geographical Location***									
Rural	44.4	32.2	9.3	1.3	12.8				
Urban	45.8	35.1	10.8	1.2	7.0				
All	45.3	34.0	10.2	1.2	9.2				

*   Education level by frequency of having a cervical smear test p < 0.05.
       Education level by "how long since last smear test?" p < 0.001.

**   p < 0.001.

†   Analysis by education level based on 1,917 (65.1 per cent) women in the sample who have ever had a cervical smear test for whom education level attained is available.
       Analysis by employment status based on 1,942 (65.2 per cent) women in the sample who have ever had a cervical smear test.

of rural women who do not know how often a woman should have a smear test contrasts with the 7 per cent of urban women falling into this category. The time elapsed since having the most recent smear test was not significantly related to geographical location.

While 8.5 per cent of women are estimated to have had an abnormal smear test, there is no significant relationship with age, medical-card status, educational experience, employment status, marital status, social class, whether a woman has had a baby or the number of babies delivered. It is interesting, however, that there is a significant relationship with geographical location, and the estimates are presented in Table 5.6. The proportion of women who have had an abnormal smear test varies from a low of 3.4 per cent in the Midland Health-Board region to a high of over 10 per

Table 5.6: Ever Had an Abnormal Cervical Smear, by Health-Board Area, and Geographical Location[†]

	Ever Had an Abnormal Cervical Smear?	
	Yes	No
Health-Board Area*	%	%
East	10.8	89.3
Midlands	3.4	96.6
Mid-West	7.6	92.5
North-East	4.5	95.5
North-West	6.0	94.0
South	8.0	92.0
South-East	10.1	89.9
West	8.8	91.2
All	8.5	91.5
Geographical Location**		
Rural	6.3	93.7
Urban	9.9	90.1
All	8.5	91.5

* $p < 0.05$.
** $p < 0.01$.
†   Analysis based on 1,942 (65.2 per cent) women in the sample who had ever had a cervical smear test.

cent in the South-East and the East. The estimate for women in urban areas is again 10 per cent compared with 6 per cent in rural areas. The 6 per cent of women who have had a family member with an abnormal smear test and the 4 per cent estimated to have had a female relative with cancer of the cervix were not found to be significantly associated with any of the demographic or geographical variables. It is worth noting, however, that the 6 per cent of women attending a gynaecologist for services other than antenatal care who had a female relative with cancer of the cervix is significantly higher than the 3 per cent of women attending who did not have a relative with this condition.

The Menopause

While the majority of women (61 per cent) consider that they have or can get adequate information on the menopause, this estimate varies significantly by age, medical-card status, employment status, geographical location and social class. Estimates regarding the adequacy of information on the menopause by age group and social class are presented in Table 5.7. Between one-half and three-quarters of women in all age groups consider that there is adequate information available on the menopause. It is probably not surprising that this proportion increases from the younger age groups to the older groups. The social-class variation in the proportion of women who do not know whether they can get adequate information on the menopause is particularly striking. While 13 per cent of women in the lower professional group fall within this category, this increases to a high of 29 per cent of women in the unskilled manual group who do not know whether adequate information on the menopause is available to them.

Over 57 per cent of medical-card holders consider information on the menopause to be adequate, compared with 62 per cent of non-medical-card holders. The 26 per cent of unemployed women who do not have enough information on the menopause is the highest proportion for all categories of employment and contrasts with the lowest estimate of 18 per cent for working women. While the proportion of women who consider that information on the menopause is adequate ranges from 57 per cent for the Western Health-Board area to 68 per cent in the South, the estimate drops to a low of 49 per cent in the Midlands.

Table 5.7: Adequacy of Information on the Menopause, Whether or Not HRT had been Taken/Would Be Considered During Menopause

Age Group*	Adequacy of Info. on Menopause?			Ever taken/are taking HRT?		Consider taking HRT during Menopause?[†]		
	Yes	*No*	*Don't Know*	*Yes*	*No*	*Yes*	*No*	*Don't Know*
	%	*%*	*%*	*%*	*%*	*%*	*%*	*%*
18–24	51.2	17.6	31.2	1.5	98.5	44.6	8.1	47.4
25–29	53.9	18.3	27.8	1.1	98.9	55.2	8.8	36.0
30–34	53.8	21.3	24.9	0.6	99.4	58.5	7.5	34.0
35–39	60.4	21.2	18.4	2.6	97.4	58.2	10.5	31.3
40–44	64.1	23.5	12.4	7.2	92.8	65.5	9.9	24.6
45–49	68.7	23.4	8.0	14.6	85.4	54.2	22.4	23.4
50–54	73.0	17.0	10.0	24.7	75.3	32.4	37.4	30.2
55–60	73.1	16.6	10.4	17.6	82.4	26.7	38.9	34.3
All	60.5	19.8	19.7	7.1	92.9	51.0	14.7	34.3
*Social Class**								
Higher Professional	65.8	16.6	17.6	9.5	90.5	63.4	15.9	20.1
Lower Professional	66.8	20.2	13.0	9.5	90.5	60.6	16.9	22.5
Other Non-Manual	62.5	19.8	17.8	6.1	93.9	52.5	13.2	34.3
Skilled Manual	61.6	21.7	16.7	10.5	89.5	50.0	17.0	33.0
Semi-skilled Manual	55.7	20.9	23.3	4.9	95.1	45.6	15.0	39.4
Unskilled Manual	49.9	20.7	29.4	3.5	96.5	33.6	17.5	49.0
All	61.4	20.1	18.5	7.3	92.7	52.1	15.4	32.6

*   p < 0.001.
†   Analysis limited to women who had never taken HRT.

For all age groups, the general practitioner is the source most women would use for information on the menopause. The symptoms most commonly associated with the menopause are hot flushes, the termination of periods and irritability. These symptoms dominate in analysis with all the demographic and geographical variables. The fact that hormone replacement therapy may be prescribed to relieve the symptoms of the menopause is known by over half the population of women. The proportion of women who do not know why hormone replacement therapy may be prescribed is a substantial 24 per cent for the population as a whole and reaches higher levels for particular population categories, including 42 per cent for 18–24 year olds and unemployed women, 35 per cent for medical-card holders and those with primary-level education only and 30 per cent for women from rural areas.

Whether or not women had actually taken hormone replacement therapy (HRT) or would consider taking HRT is presented by age group and social class in Table 5.7. As expected, the utilisation of HRT is mainly found among women aged 45 and over. Notwithstanding the persistence of certain controversies regarding the use of HRT, it is interesting that HRT use has only reached a high of one-quarter for the 50–54 age group (Klein and Dumble, 1994; Worcester and Whatley, 1992). Attitudes to taking HRT are clearly related to age, with estimates of between one-half and two-thirds of women aged between 25 and 45 positively oriented to taking HRT during the menopause.

Table 5.7 shows that around three times as many women in the higher professional, lower professional and skilled manual classes have ever taken HRT when compared with estimates for women in the unskilled manual group. There is a strong social-class effect on whether or not women would consider taking HRT during the menopause. The high estimate of 63 per cent of women in the higher professional group who would consider taking HRT during the menopause declines through the social-class hierarchy to a low of 34 per cent in the unskilled manual group. The social-class gradient for those who do not know if they would take HRT during the menopause is in the opposite direction beginning with 20 per cent of women in the higher professional group and increasing to a high of 49 per cent in the unskilled manual group.

While the experience of having taken HRT is not related to medical-card status, Table 5.8 shows that at 54 per cent, a higher proportion of women without medical cards say they would consider taking HRT during the menopause compared with 44 per cent for women with medical cards. The 39 per cent of medical-card holders who do not know whether they would take HRT is somewhat higher than the 33 per cent estimated for women without medical cards.

Table 5.8: Information on Osteoporosis, People Noted as Being at Risk from Osteoporosis, Avoiding Osteoporosis and Preference for HRT, by Medical-Card Status

	Medical-Card Status		
	Yes	No	All
What is Osteoporosis?*	%	%	%
Thinning of the bones[†]	60.1	77.6	72.3
Other/Don't Know	39.9	22.4	27.7
*People Most at Risk from Osteoporosis?**			
Young Women	1.0	0.9	0.9
Middle-Aged/Older Women[†]	44.4	56.0	52.5
Children	0.4	0.4	0.4
Men	0.1	0.2	0.2
Old People[†]	21.5	18.9	19.7
Other	4.2	6.7	5.9
Don't Know	28.5	16.8	20.3
*Causes of Osteoporosis**			
Lack of oestrogen due to menopause[†]	9.8	13.8	12.6
Lack of calcium in bones[†]	46.4	57.8	54.5
Arthritis	2.9	1.6	2.0
Lack of exercise	2.7	6.2	5.2
Overweight	2.2	0.9	1.3
Other	5.8	4.8	5.1
Don't Know	30.2	14.9	19.3
*How Can Osteoporosis Be Avoided?**			
Taking HRT	9.7	13.3	12.3
Taking exercise	8.8	13.5	12.2
Taking a calcium-high diet	46.3	55.7	53.1
Other	3.4	3.6	3.5
Don't Know	31.8	13.9	18.8
Consider Taking HRT During Menopause?[†][†]			
Yes	44.3	53.5	50.7
No	16.6	14.0	14.7
Don't Know	39.1	32.6	34.6

*   p < 0.001.
†   Most appropriate response.
††   Analysis limited to women who have never taken HRT.

Experience of taking HRT and attitudes to taking HRT by educational experience and employment status are addressed in Table 5.9 While the estimate for the proportion of women who have taken HRT drops from a high of 11 per cent for women with primary education to 9 per cent for university graduates, the trend is in the opposite direction in terms of attitudes to taking HRT. The 45 per cent of women with primary education only who would consider taking HRT contrasts with a high of 60 per cent for university graduates. At 10 per cent, women engaged in home duties have the highest estimate for utilisation of HRT by employment status. In addition, over half the women in this category or working full-time, and 61 per cent of those working part-time, would

Table 5.9: Ever Taken/Are Taking HRT, and Consider Taking HRT During Menopause, by Education Level and Employment Status

	Ever taken / Are taking HRT?		*Consider taking HRT During Menopause*[†]		
	Yes	*No*	*Yes*	*No*	*Don't Know*
Education Level*	%	%	%	%	%
Primary Cert/Lower	10.9	89.1	44.6	21.6	33.8
Inter/Group/Junior Cert	6.5	93.5	47.3	15.9	36.8
Leaving Cert/Matric	5.3	94.7	54.2	10.7	35.1
Qualification from RTC etc.	4.5	95.5	57.8	10.8	31.3
University Qualification	8.5	91.5	60.4	16.6	23.0
All	7.0	92.9	51.1	14.8	34.1
Employment Status*					
Working Full-time	4.0	96.0	52.5	12.1	35.4
Working Part-time	8.9	91.1	61.4	10.9	27.8
Unemployed	3.1	96.9	40.7	12.0	47.3
Home Duties	10.1	89.9	50.3	18.5	31.2
Students/Retired/Ill/Disabled	3.3	96.7	48.1	9.6	42.3
All	7.1	92.9	51.0	14.7	34.3

*   p < 0.001.
†   Analysis limited to women who have never taken HRT.

consider using HRT during the menopause. A positive approach to taking HRT is also put forward by 55 per cent of women from urban areas compared with 46 per cent for those from rural areas.

A logistic regression model was fitted for the variable whether or not HRT had been taken by women aged between 45 and 60. Urban/rural location was found to be confounded with Health-Board area of residence. Age and the Health-Board area of residence variable were found to be significant and the parameter estimates are presented in Table A6. The negative intercept indicates that women aged between 45 and 60 are generally more likely not to have taken HRT, though from amongst this group women aged 50–54 would be the most likely to have taken HRT. The variation by Health-Board area is interesting with uptake shown to be highest in the East and the South and lowest in the West and the South East. The estimation of the combined effect of these variables from these results provides an interesting illustration. The probability of women in the 50–54 age group in the Southern Health-Board area having taken HRT is estimated at .29, which contrasts with the probability of .08 estimated for women aged 45–49 in the Western Health-Board area.

An additional logistic regression model estimated for whether or not women in the 45–60 age group would take HRT also found that age was significant. Medical-card status and maternal status were confounded within the age variable. The results of this analysis show that younger women are more likely to consider taking HRT during the menopause. The strong effect of age on this variable is illustrated by the finding that an estimated 54 per cent of women aged 45–49 would consider taking HRT, compared with the estimate of 29 per cent for women aged 55–60.

Self-Examination of Breasts

The frequency with which women may or m~ ~ not undertake self-examination of their breasts is significantly associated with age, medical-card status, social class, educational experience, employment status and health-board area of residence. An analysis by age group of factors associated with self-examination of breasts is presented in Table 5.10. With regard to those women who report performing self-examination of breasts frequently, the proportion increases from 12 per cent for the 18–24 age group to 30 per cent for the 40–44 year olds, with a subsequent decline for those aged

50 and over. While an estimated 58 per cent of women in the 18–24 group report never performing self-examination of breasts, this falls to a low of 29 per cent for the 35–44 group and rises again to 40 per cent for those aged 55–60.

Table 5.10: Frequency and Timing of Breast Self-Examination, Together with Preference for Who Conducts Breast Examination, by Age Group

Age Group*	Frequency of Performing Self-Examination of Breasts			Best Time of the Month for Breast Examination			Preference for Who Conducts Breast Examination		
	Frequently	*Occasionally*	*Never*	*Week Following Period[†]*	*Other*	*Don't Know*	*Male Doctor*	*Female Doctor*	*Don't Mind / Other*
	%	%	%	%	%	%	%	%	%
18–24	11.8	29.8	58.4	27.1	15.8	57.1	1.5	52.5	46.1
25–29	23.9	40.3	35.8	41.8	18.1	40.1	1.5	49.5	49.0
30–34	23.6	40.7	35.8	42.5	16.9	40.6	3.0	40.3	56.7
35–39	26.3	44.9	28.9	51.9	19.2	28.9	2.7	44.8	52.5
40–44	30.2	40.5	29.4	48.2	20.6	31.2	2.4	34.3	63.3
45–49	29.6	36.3	34.1	53.8	15.5	30.7	3.7	36.2	60.1
50–54	24.8	39.6	35.6	43.0	18.2	38.8	3.7	33.9	62.4
55–60	25.6	34.6	39.9	33.3	11.8	54.8	1.7	37.3	61.0
All	23.4	37.9	38.7	41.6	17.0	41.3	2.4	42.5	55.1

* $p < 0.001$.
† Most appropriate response.

Given that regular breast self-examination is recommended for the early detection of abnormalities, it is cause for serious concern that 39 per cent of women say that they never examine their breasts. The variation by social class for this group of women is clearly in evidence from Table 5.11 which shows the 29 per cent of women in the higher and lower professional groups who never conduct breast self-examination increasing to 45 and 43 per cent, respectively, for women in the semi-skilled and unskilled manual groups. The social class variation in the occasional conduct of breast self-examination moves in the other direction, declining from a high of 43 per cent for the higher professional group to 32 per cent of women in the unskilled manual group. This table also shows that non-medical-card holders are generally more likely to conduct breast self-examination than are medical-card holders.

Table 5.11: Frequency and Timing of Breast Self-Examination, by Social Class and Medical-Card Status

Social Class*	Frequency of Performing Self-Examination of Breasts			Best Time of the Month for Breast Examination		
	Frequently	Occasionally	Never	Week Following Period[†]	Other	Don't Know
	%	%	%	%	%	%
Higher Professional	28.0	43.1	28.9	54.9	15.4	29.8
Lower Professional	27.5	42.8	29.7	50.8	18.7	30.6
Other Non-Manual	23.4	40.4	36.2	40.2	17.6	42.2
Skilled Manual	25.3	38.2	36.5	45.9	14.3	39.8
Semi-skilled Manual	20.6	34.0	45.4	36.8	17.6	45.6
Unskilled Manual	24.9	31.7	43.4	30.8	18.2	51.1
All	24.5	39.0	36.5	43.2	17.2	39.6
*Medical-Card Status***						
Yes	23.6	34.0	42.5	37.5	16.2	46.3
No	23.8	39.6	36.6	44.0	16.8	39.2
All	23.7	37.9	38.4	42.0	16.6	41.3

* p < 0.001.
** Medical-card status by "Frequency of Performing Self-Examination of Breasts": p < 0.005.
Medical-card status by "Best Time of the Month for Breast Examination": p < 0.001.
† Most appropriate response.

Frequency of performing self-examination of breasts is presented in Table 5.12 for different levels of educational experience and employment status. The estimate for those performing this examination occasionally is shown to increase within increasing levels of education, while the opposite is true for women who never perform breast self-examination. Close to 44 per cent of women with primary education never conduct this examination,

Table 5.12: Frequency of Performing Self-Examination of Breasts, and Best Time of Month for Breast Examination, by Education Level and Employment Status

	Frequency of Performing Self-Examination of Breasts			Best Time of Month for Breast Examination		
	Frequently	*Occasionally*	*Never*	*Week Following Period[†]*	*Other*	*Don't know*
Education Level*	%	%	%	%	%	%
Primary Cert/Lower	26.8	29.5	43.7	37.5	15.8	46.7
Inter/Group/Junior Cert	23.9	40.4	35.7	41.9	18.0	40.1
Leaving Cert/Matric	23.1	39.2	37.7	45.3	15.5	39.2
Qualification from RTC, etc.	18.6	42.8	38.6	33.4	26.5	40.1
University Qualification	18.5	45.3	36.2	41.6	18.8	39.6
All	23.5	38.1	38.4	41.8	17.0	41.2
Employment Status*						
Working Full-time	18.9	41.1	40.1	40.3	17.6	42.1
Working Part-time	24.7	40.0	35.3	46.9	18.1	34.9
Unemployed	20.1	30.8	49.1	32.5	18.2	49.3
Home Duties	29.3	37.5	33.2	46.0	16.4	37.6
Student/Retired/Ill/Disabled	10.1	29.9	60.1	24.1	16.9	59.1
All	23.4	37.9	38.7	41.6	17.0	41.3

*   p < 0.001.
†   Most appropriate response.

compared with 36 per cent of women with university qualifications. Women engaged in home duties show the highest estimate
for performing breast self-examination frequently, while working
women are estimated to have the highest probability of performing this examination occasionally. With an estimate of 60 per cent,
women in the category that includes students, the retired and the
ill/disabled have the highest proportion of women who never perform self-examination of breasts.

For those women who did not undertake self-examination of
their breasts, most have no particular reason for not performing
the examination. One-third of women aged between 45 and 54
years don't because they are afraid of what they might find. This
is the population group for which this anxiety is strongest. Given
the risk factors for women in this age group, these concerns would
seem to warrant specific attention where policy initiatives in this
area are being considered.

With regard to the best time of the month for this examination,
the information presented in Table 5.10 indicates that women in
the 45–49 age category are the best informed, as over half the
group are estimated to know the best time and 31 per cent fall
into the "don't know" category. This contrasts with the findings for
the 18–24 age group where the corresponding estimates are 27
per cent and 57 per cent, respectively. Table 5.11 shows that over
one in every two women in the higher and lower professional
groups know that the week following a period is the best time for
breast self-examination, compared with just 31 per cent of women
in the unskilled manual group. Only 38 per cent of medical-card
holders know the best time of the month to conduct this examination, compared with 44 per cent of non-medical-card holders.

The estimates by educational experience and employment
status presented in Table 5.12 show that women with leaving
certificate, working women and those engaged in home duties are
more likely to know the best time of the month for breast self-
examination. The women who are most likely to respond "don't
know" to this question are those with primary education only, the
unemployed, students, the retired and the ill/disabled.

With regard to the estimated preference for who conducts a
breast examination, Table 5.10 shows that a very small proportion in all age groups have a preference for a male doctor. The
preference for a female doctor is highest for women under 40,
after which the estimate is over 60 per cent for those who "don't

mind" who performs the examination.

Over 13 per cent of the female population are estimated to have had a female relative with breast cancer. Among women who have had a relative with this condition, breast self-examination is estimated to be undertaken frequently by 28 per cent, occasionally by 35 per cent, with 37 per cent reportedly never undertaking this examination. For women who do not have a relative with breast cancer, 23 per cent undertake breast self-examination frequently while 39 per cent and 38 per cent, respectively, undertake breast self-examination either occasionally or not at all. Having a female relative with breast cancer is significantly associated with the approach taken to performing self-examination of breasts.

Common Medical Conditions Experienced by Women

Osteoporosis

According to the information presented in Table 5.13, an estimated one-fifth to one-third of women across the different age groups do not understand that osteoporosis is a gradual thinning of the bones. At 56 per cent, the proportion of women with primary education who understand the nature of the condition of osteoporosis contrasts with an estimate of 93 per cent for women with university qualifications. The groups most at risk for osteoporosis do, however, seem to be generally correctly identified as middle-aged/older women and old people across the different age groups and for different levels of educational experience and employment status. Table 5.13 shows some variation by age group as middle-aged/older women are seen to be at risk by an estimated 42 per cent of 18–24-year-olds compared with higher estimates of 61 per cent for the 35–39 group. This reaches a high of 73 per cent for women with university education. The proportion of women who cannot identify the groups most at risk from osteoporosis is quite substantial and is estimated to be about one-third for women who are unemployed or who have primary education, and ranges between 15 and 30 per cent for the different age groups.

Knowledge about osteoporosis by medical-card status is reported in Table 5.8. At 60 per cent and 78 per cent, respectively, there is quite a substantial difference between women with and without medical cards in their understanding of the condition of

Table 5.13: Information on Osteoporosis, People Noted as being at Risk from Osteoporosis, Causes of Osteoporosis and Approaches to Avoid Osteoporosis, by Age Group

	Age Group								
	18–24	*25–29*	*30–34*	*35–39*	*40–44*	*45–49*	*50–54*	*55–60*	*All*
*What is Osteoporosis?**	%	%	%	%	%	%	%	%	%
Thinning of the bones[†]	67.6	63.4	71.3	76.7	78.4	79.6	78.3	72.4	72.6
Other/Don't know	32.4	36.6	28.7	23.3	21.6	20.4	21.7	27.7	27.4
*People most at risk from Osteoporosis**									
Young Women	2.3	0.6	0.9	0.6	0.9	0.3	0.3	0.6	1.0
Middle-Aged/ Older Women[†]	42.0	47.1	52.8	61.4	55.6	59.8	55.2	58.5	52.9
Children	0.2	0.8	0.6	0.9	0.0	0.2	0.8	0.0	0.4
Men	0.2	0.0	0.2	0.4	0.0	0.3	0.0	0.3	0.2
Old People[+]	25.2	18.0	18.8	17.8	18.3	18.1	15.2	18.7	19.4
Other	6.0	4.9	6.9	4.0	5.9	6.4	9.1	6.3	6.0
Don't Know	24.1	28.6	19.8	14.9	19.2	14.9	19.4	15.6	20.1
*Causes of Osteoporosis**									
Lack of oestrogen caused by menopause[†]	9.2	8.2	8.8	13.6	13.4	18.0	17.3	16.9	12.6
Lack of calcium in bones[†]	54.5	53.2	59.7	58.4	55.7	53.8	52.4	50.2	54.7
Arthritis	2.4	1.0	2.0	2.2	1.6	1.6	2.2	2.5	1.9
Lack of exercise[†]	4.5	3.6	4.0	5.9	5.8	7.0	4.3	6.0	5.1
Overweight	0.8	1.6	1.0	1.5	1.3	1.0	1.1	2.1	1.3
Other	7.0	4.7	3.7	4.0	5.6	5.3	6.0	5.1	5.3
Don't Know	22.6	27.7	20.9	14.4	16.7	13.4	17.0	17.1	19.1
*How can Osteoporosis be avoided?**									
Taking HRT	7.6	9.2	9.9	11.6	13.8	17.1	18.0	16.3	12.3
Taking exercise	11.7	8.6	10.7	15.2	13.0	14.3	13.0	12.1	12.3
Taking a calcium-high diet	54.2	50.8	56.3	55.6	54.0	52.6	47.8	50.7	53.1
Other	4.0	3.5	3.9	3.8	23.4	3.7	3.7	3.7	3.7
Don't Know	22.6	27.9	19.1	13.7	15.8	12.3	17.5	17.3	18.6

*   p < 0.001.

†   Most appropriate response.

osteoporosis. This difference is also in evidence for the identification of the population groups most at risk for this condition. While 56 per cent of non-medical-card holders identified middle aged/ older women as being a high-risk group, this contrasts with the estimated 44 per cent among the medical-card holders for this category. Approximately 29 per cent of medical-card holders do not know the answer to the question of who is most at risk from osteoporosis, compared with 17 per cent of non-medical-card holders.

Table 5.13 shows that over half the population of women across all age groups recognise that lack of calcium is a cause of osteoporosis. Lack of knowledge about the cause of this condition is as high as 34 per cent among women with primary education and 30 per cent among unemployed women. The proportion of women in this category decreases with increasing age from 28 per cent for those aged 25–29 to 13 per cent for the 45–49 age group. The trend is in the opposite direction for those who consider lack of oestrogen caused by the menopause to be a causal factor, with the estimate increasing from 9 per cent for the 18–24 group to 17 per cent for those aged 50 and over.

Table 5.8 shows that 56 per cent of non-medical-card holders consider lack of calcium to be a cause of osteoporosis, which contrasts with the 46 per cent estimated for medical-card holders. With an estimate of 10 per cent, medical-card holders are also less likely to consider lack of oestrogen resulting from the menopause as a causal factor, though the corresponding estimate is just 13 per cent for non-medical-card holders.

Taking a calcium-high diet is the most widely known approach to avoiding osteoporosis across all levels of employment status, educational experience and age groups. Table 5.13 shows that a substantial proportion of women in all age groups do not know how osteoporosis can be avoided. Over one-third of women who are unemployed or with primary-level education also fall into this category. Table 5.8 shows that an estimated 32 per cent of medical-card holders do not know how osteoporosis can be avoided, compared with just 14 per cent of non-medical-card holders. Taking a calcium-high diet was the predominant response to this question among both groups.

Unavoidable Leakage of Urine

Just over 25 per cent of women are estimated to have experienced unavoidable leakage of urine at some time in their life. Variation by age in the experience of this condition is presented in Table 5.14. A clear pattern is evident here with between 29 and 35 per cent of the women over 30 estimated to have experienced unavoidable leakage of urine. For those women who have had this experience, close to 40 per cent of those aged 40 and over are estimated to consider that unavoidable leakage of urine continues to be a problem for them. Even for the younger age groups, the current experience of this problem is estimated at 28 per cent for those aged 30–34. Over half those who have experienced this problem have sought help, with two-thirds of this group going to the general practitioner for assistance. The majority of those who did not seek help said that they had learned to live with the condition.

Table 5.14: Experience of Unavoidable Leakage of Urine, by Age Group

	Ever Experienced Leakage of Urine?*		*Leaking of Urine a Problem Now?**[†]	
	Yes	*No*	*Yes*	*No*
Age Group	*%*	*%*	*%*	*%*
18–24	8.7	91.3	24.1	5.9
25–30	17.5	82.5	17.9	82.1
30–34	29.2	70.8	28.0	72.0
35–39	28.7	71.3	23.4	76.6
40–44	34.5	65.5	40.4	59.6
45–49	31.9	68.2	42.8	57.2
50–54	35.8	64.2	37.4	62.6
55–60	29.5	70.5	43.6	56.4
All	25.1	74.9	33.1	66.9

* $p < 0.001$.
†   Analysis based on 750 (25.1 per cent) women in the sample who had experienced unavoidable leakage of urine.

Conclusion

The information presented here provides some very interesting insights into attitudes to and utilisation of gynaecology services by Irish women. At a general level, however, the findings are cause for concern as they reveal large gaps in information and knowledge among women regarding important practices for the promotion and maintenance of good health. Too many women do not know when they should have a smear test or when to conduct breast self-examination or how to avoid osteoporosis. Even when women provide the correct answer to many of these questions, the practice too often falls short of the recommended standard.

The importance of screening as a means of reducing the incidence of breast cancer and cervical cancer among women has long been emphasised in the health promotion literature and in the health promotion strategies pursued by the Department of Health (1995c). The recently published discussion document on developing a policy for women's health notes the commitment of the Minister for Health to a phased expansion of a breast-cancer screening programme for women within specified age groups (Department of Health, 1995a). The discussion document also notes that a major impediment to the development of a national screening programme for cervical cancer is the absence of a population register for women (Department of Health, 1995a). The fact that more than one woman in every three has never had a smear test and never conducts breast self-examination is, however, cause for serious concern. The absence of such a register should not in any way impede the pursuit of targeted health promotion strategies aimed at making more women better informed about the importance of such practices as breast self-examination and regular cervical smear tests for the maintenance of good health. Given that osteoporosis is such a common condition among women, the level of ignorance about how it can be avoided is somewhat surprising. It would therefore be advisable to include the dissemination of information on the causes of osteoporosis and ways to avoid the condition in any strategy aimed at improving the knowledge and the pursuit of health promotion practices among women.

6

Having a Baby:
Antenatal and Postnatal Experience, Maternity Leave, Family Size and Parenting Skills

Introduction

For the majority of Irish women, childbirth takes place in the hospital. The hospital is therefore an important source for both antenatal and postnatal care and this chapter addresses questions regarding the acceptability and preferences for hospital-based, childbirth-related services for Irish women. In addition, the issues of the availability and extent of maternity leave, the desired and actual family size and acquisition of parenting skills are also addressed.

The movement of childbirth from the home to the hospital has been associated with the development of programmes intending to prepare expectant mothers for the less familiar hospital environment. These programmes have grown into the antenatal classes, which have come to incorporate a wide range of objectives, including the provision of education on the pregnancy and birth process, the development of techniques to assist coping with labour, physical preparation for delivery, knowledge of baby care and breast-feeding and preparation for the transition to parenthood (Chalmers and McIntyre, 1994). As attendance at antenatal classes has been shown in previous studies to improve birth outcomes, this study is concerned with assessing the pattern of attendance at these classes among Irish mothers (Stewart et al., 1993). In addition, opinions were elicited on the health services received antenatally and postnatally and the extent to which these services were considered to be an adequate preparation for motherhood.

The experiences of the two-thirds of Irish women who have ever had a baby are the focus of interest here. As more mothers continue to participate in the labour force, issues like maternity leave, the availability of child-care facilities and family size have become increasingly important. While the introduction of benefits like maternity leave has meant that motherhood and labour-force participation are not necessarily mutually exclusive, it was considered timely to assess the perceived adequacy of the benefits available to working mothers.

For women who have had a baby, the mean number of babies delivered is 3.3, with the first baby being born to women at an average age of 24.5 years and the most recent baby born to women at an average age of 31.2 years. Only 5 per cent of women are estimated to have given birth at home intentionally, while 14 per cent of those who did not give birth at home would have liked to do so.

An estimated 76 per cent of mothers believe that tests should be available in Irish hospitals to show prior to birth whether a baby has any abnormality. Close to 31 per cent of mothers attended antenatal classes in preparation for childbirth.[1] Approximately three out of four mothers attended for classes in the hospital, while 17 per cent attended on a private basis. The reasons cited most frequently by the two-thirds of mothers who did not attend antenatal classes were the fact that none were available at the time (18 per cent), the classes were too far away (17 per cent), they did not think they were of any use (15 per cent), they had done them before (13 per cent) or they had no time (11 per cent).

Antenatal care was received by over half (57 per cent) the mothers in the public hospital clinic, with one-quarter attending the private clinic or the doctor's rooms. While 96 per cent of mothers felt that they had enough time with the midwife during antenatal visits, this dropped to a level of 78 per cent with regard to time with the doctor. The same doctor/midwife was seen by 62 per cent of mothers during antenatal visits, though 70 per cent prefer to see the same service-providers at each visit. At 83 per cent, the

---

[1]   All survey questions and results reported relating to ante and postnatal care relate to the last baby delivered to the respondent.

majority of mothers felt that they had enough privacy during the antenatal visit. Over 84 per cent of mothers felt that the antenatal classes had prepared them adequately or very well for childbirth. Partners attended the antenatal classes with just one out of every four mothers.

Taking time off for antenatal care presented a problem at work for 5 per cent of mothers. Mornings and afternoons were the times when 48 per cent and 44 per cent of mothers, respectively, attended the antenatal clinic. Similar estimates are reported for the times which mothers consider most convenient for these clinics. While the majority of mothers felt that doctors and nurses showed sufficient interest in their concerns during antenatal visits, 17 per cent felt that the interest shown by doctors was not sufficient and 11 per cent considered that sufficient interest was not shown by the nurses.

The average postnatal stay in hospital was estimated at five days. While 82 per cent of mothers considered that this was adequate, the other 18 per cent would prefer a stay of, on average, seven days. Close to 14 per cent of mothers did not think that they were adequately prepared to go home with their baby and over 38 per cent of this group would have liked further support from the public health nurse. While over half the mothers never felt depressed following childbirth, more than one in every three mothers (38 per cent) had "baby blues" and 11 per cent had postnatal depression. After returning home, over half the mothers considered that they received most help from their partner, with 22 per cent specifying a parent as an important source of support. For two-thirds of mothers, there was no change in their relationship with their partners following the arrival of a new baby and 81 per cent felt that their partners did not feel neglected.

The Antenatal and Postnatal Experience of Mothers

Antenatal Education

The findings regarding antenatal education presented here relate specifically to the birth of the woman's last baby. Despite the fact that attendance at hospital antenatal classes is free, only 31 per cent of mothers attended antenatal classes prior to the birth of their last baby. While this estimate increased to 55 per cent for women having their first baby, the estimate declined to 41 per cent for the birth of the second baby and continued to decline for

subsequent babies. While age, medical-card status, education experience, employment status and geographical location were significantly associated with attendance for antenatal education in
the bivariate analyses, the multivariate analysis found that employment status was confounded within age, urban/rural location
was confounded within health-board area of residence, and social
class was confounded within level of education.

Between 40 and 50 per cent of mothers aged between 25 and
39 participated in antenatal classes. Participation by those in the
18–24 group was estimated at the low level of 34 per cent. While
just 19 per cent of medical-card holders are estimated to have attended antenatal classes, this contrasts with the estimate of 36 per
cent for non-medical-card holders. It is clear from Table 6.1 that the
probability of attending antenatal classes increases with higher
levels of education. Just 18 per cent of mothers with a primary-
level education attended antenatal classes, compared with 53 per
cent of mothers with a university qualification. The variation by
health board shown in Table 6.1 is quite striking. While the East
and the North West record attendances of 39 per cent, participation in the other health-board areas ranges from 22 per cent to 27
per cent.

To advance the understanding of the multivariate effect on
participation in antenatal classes, a logistic regression model was
estimated. The results of this analysis presented in Table A7, Appendix 3, show the effect of age, medical-card status, education
level and health-board area of residence on whether or not women
attended antenatal classes. This analysis shows that mothers in
general are more likely not to have attended antenatal classes. As
age increases, the probability of attendance at these classes is
shown to decrease. While medical-card holders are less likely to
attend for antenatal classes, the trend for education level indicates that the probability of uptake increases with increasing
levels of education. Residence in the Eastern Health-Board region
is shown to have a strong positive effect on the probability of attendance at classes, relative to the other health-board areas. An
illustration of the effect of these results is presented in Table 6.2.
This table shows that while 69 per cent of mothers aged 30–34 with
a Leaving Certificate education, living in the Eastern Health-Board
area, are likely to attend antenatal classes, this drops to 18 per cent
for mothers aged 35–39 with a medical card and an Intermediate
Certificate education, living in the North Eastern Health Board.

Table 6.1: Attendance at Antenatal Classes, by Education Level, and Health-Board Area[†]

	Attended Antenatal Classes	
	Yes	No
*Education Level**	%	%
Primary Cert/Lower	17.5	82.5
Inter/Group/Junior Cert	28.3	71.7
Leaving Cert/Matric	39.3	60.8
Qualification from RTC, etc.	49.3	50.7
University Qualification	52.6	47.4
All	30.8	69.2
*Health-Board Area**		
East	39.3	60.7
Midland	21.7	78.3
Mid-West	24.2	75.8
North-East	25.2	74.8
North-West	39.1	60.9
South	24.4	75.6
South-East	27.2	72.8
West	23.1	76.9
All	30.9	69.1

* $p < 0.001$.

†   Analysis by education level based on 1922 (64.5 per cent) women in the sample who have had a baby and for whom education level attained is available.
Analysis by Health Board based on 1939 (65.1 per cent) women in the sample who have had a baby.

The centre of choice for antenatal classes was not significantly related to age but was significantly related to medical-card status, educational experience, employment status and geographical location. Table 6.3 shows that while the hospital was the venue most frequently chosen for antenatal classes, there was some variation in attendances at health centres and at private centres. The 21 per cent of non-medical-card holders estimated to have

Table 6.2: Estimation of the Likelihood of Mothers with Specified Characteristics of Attending Antenatal Classes for the Birth of Their Last Baby

Mothers with Specified Characteristics	*Likelihood of Attending Antenatal Classes*
1. Age 30–34 Leaving Cert No medical card Eastern Health Board	0.69
2. Age 35–39 Inter Cert With medical card North Eastern Health Board	0.18
3. Age 40–44 University education With medical card Western Health Board	0.22
4. Age 40–44 Leaving Cert No medical card Eastern Health Board	0.47
5. Age 50–54 Primary education No medical card Southern Health Board	0.10

participated in antenatal education on a private basis, contrasts with the 4 per cent estimated for medical-card holders. Over 16 per cent of mothers with medical cards attended health centres for antenatal classes compared with 7 per cent of non-medical-card holders.

It is interesting to note from Table 6.3 that attendance at hospital antenatal classes drops from a high of 90 per cent for mothers with primary education only to a low of 53 per cent for those with university qualifications. The opposite trend is in evidence for attendance at private clinics, where the estimate increases from 3 per cent at the lowest level of educational attainment to a high of 34 per cent for mothers with university education. One in every four mothers working full-time and 15 per cent of mothers working part-time or engaged in home duties receive private antenatal education. The hospital is still the most popular choice of antenatal education across all employment categories.

Table 6.3: Where Antenatal Classes Were Attended, by Education Level, Employment Status, and Medical-Card Status[†]

| | Where Attended Antenatal Classes | | | |
| | Hospital | Health Centre | Privately | Other |
Education Level*	%	%	%	%
Primary Cert/Lower	89.6	7.5	3.0	0.0
Inter/Group/Junior Cert	75.9	11.8	11.2	1.1
Leaving Cert/Matric	70.4	7.1	21.5	1.0
Qualification from RTC, etc.	69.6	2.8	27.6	0.0
University Qualification	52.9	11.7	33.7	1.6
All	73.3	8.8	17.1	0.9
*Employment Status**				
Working Full-time	62.2	8.3	26.3	3.2
Working Part-time	76.5	8.4	15.1	0.0
Unemployed	91.2	8.8	0.0	0.0
Home Duties	76.4	9.0	14.6	0.0
Student/Retired/Ill/Disabled	100.0	0.0	0.0	0.0
All	73.3	8.7	17.1	0.9
*Medical-Card Status**				
Yes	79.0	16.4	3.8	0.8
No	70.9	7.0	21.1	1.0
All	72.8	9.1	17.2	0.9

* $p < 0.001$.
† Analysis based on mothers who had attended antenatal classes in preparation for the birth of their last baby, i.e. 30.9 per cent of mothers.

The variation, shown in Table 6.4, in where mothers attend for antenatal classes, by health board, is interesting and may indicate

availability as well as preferences. While 87 per cent of mothers in
the East went to the hospital for classes, this contrasted with the
estimate of 34 per cent for the South East where attendance at
the health centres and private clinics was highest. Private clinics
were also attended by over one-third of mothers in the North East
and the South, while attendance in this category was just over 8
per cent for the East and the North West. In general, the participation in private antenatal education was estimated at 28 per
cent for rural women and 11 per cent for urban women. Women in
urban areas were more likely to attend the hospital, with a participation rate of 81 per cent, compared with 58 per cent for
women in rural areas.

**Table 6.4: Where Antenatal Classes Were Attended,
by Health-Board Area, and Geographical Location[†]**

	Where Attended Antenatal Classes			
	Hospital	Health Centre	Privately	Other
Health-Board Area*	%	%	%	%
East	86.6	4.6	8.1	0.7
Midland	71.0	5.6	23.5	0.0
Mid-West	81.1	0.0	18.9	0.0
North-East	58.9	5.3	35.7	0.0
North-West	67.2	20.1	8.7	4.0
South	59.1	5.4	34.0	1.4
South-East	34.2	27.3	38.6	0.0
West	68.4	19.4	12.2	0.0
All	73.3	8.7	17.1	0.9
Geographical Location*				
Rural	58.0	12.1	28.3	1.6
Urban	81.3	6.9	11.3	0.5
All	73.3	8.7	17.1	0.9

*　p < 0.001.
†　Analysis based on mothers who had attended antenatal classes in preparation for the birth of their last baby, i.e. 30.9 per cent of mothers.

While partners attended antenatal classes with just over one
in every four mothers, this varied by age, medical-card status,

educational experience, employment status and social class. About one-third of women aged between 25 and 39 were accompanied by their partners. A similar estimate was found for women working full-time and women with Leaving Certificate or university qualifications. The partners of just 15 per cent of medical-card holders attended the classes, compared with 29 per cent for non-medical-card holders. Partners of women with RTC qualifications showed the highest level of participation in antenatal classes at 54 per cent. While the partners of 36 per cent of women in the higher professional group attended antenatal classes, this declined for the other social classes to 17 per cent for the skilled manual group and zero for those in the unskilled manual group.

The level of satisfaction with the antenatal classes attended was generally high, as over 84 per cent of participants believed that the classes prepared them very well/adequately for the birth. Level of satisfaction as it relates to the centre where the classes were received is presented in Table 6.5. The highest estimate in the very well/adequate category is 91 per cent and is found for those attending for classes on a private basis. The hospital ranks third with an estimate of 84 per cent, and 73 per cent are estimated to consider that the antenatal classes received at the health centre prepared them very well/adequately for childbirth.

Table 6.5: Adequacy of Preparation for Birth, by Antenatal Classes According to Where Classes Were Attended[†]

	Adequacy of Preparation for Birth by Antenatal Classes			
*Where Attended Antenatal Classes**	*Very Adequate* %	*Adequate* %	*Inadequate* %	*Very Inadequate* %
Hospital	37.1	46.9	10.5	5.6
Health Centre	33.8	39.6	20.4	6.2
Privately	52.8	38.2	7.0	2.0
Other	54.5	27.0	18.5	0.0
All	39.6	44.7	10.8	5.0

* $p < 0.05$.

†   Analysis based on mothers who had attended antenatal classes in preparation for the birth of their last baby, i.e. 30.9 per cent of mothers.

It has been previously noted that the most frequently cited reasons for not attending antenatal classes included the fact that the classes were not available, were too far away, were not thought to be of any use, had been done previously or that there was no time to do the classes. The specific reasons put forward by the mothers who did not do the classes varied by age, medical-card status, educational experience, geographical location, employment status and social class.[2] The fact that the classes were "too far away" was specified by a high of 21 per cent of mothers in the 25–30 age group. Close to 21 per cent of mothers with medical cards also considered this to be a problem, compared with 15 per cent of non-medical-card holders. Over one-quarter of mothers in the 18–24 group did not think that the classes were of any use, while more than one-fifth of those aged 30–39 had done them before. This reason was also specified by 18 per cent of non-medical-card holders, compared with 6 per cent of mothers with medical cards.

The higher the level of educational experience, the less likely mothers are to consider antenatal classes not to be of any use. While this response was given by 18 per cent of those with primary-level education only, this compared with just 4 per cent for university graduates. The contrasting trend is in evidence for the response that the classes had been taken previously, with 5 per cent of those with primary education in this group compared with 29 per cent for mothers with a university qualification.

The most frequently cited reasons by mothers working full-time for being unable to attend antenatal classes were that they were too far away (17 per cent), they had no time (16 per cent), or that there were none available (16 per cent). At 22 per cent, the reason most frequently cited by the unemployed for not attending classes was that they had done them before. For mothers engaged in home duties, the most likely reasons for not attending classes were that they had no time (18 per cent) or that there were none available (19 per cent). For mothers in the higher and lower professional groups, the most frequently cited reason for non-attendance was that they had done them before. One in five mothers in the skilled manual and semi-skilled manual groups did not attend these classes because, for those in the first category they were too far away, and for those in the second category they

---

[2]   The responses to the question why antenatal classes were not attended were not mutually exclusive so respondents may have given more than one reason for non-attendance.

were considered too costly. For mothers in the other non-manual and unskilled manual groups, one in five said that antenatal classes were not available.

The availability and location of classes were important factors determining uptake by mothers on a geographical basis. For those in rural areas, the most frequently cited reasons for not attending classes were that they were too far away (27 per cent) or that they were not available (21 per cent). This contrasts with the pattern in evidence for women from urban areas where they were more likely to consider that the classes were not of any use (20 per cent) or that they had done them before (18 per cent). Close to one-third of the mothers in the health-board regions of the Midlands, the North West and the South East put forward the reasons that antenatal classes were not available. Over one-fifth of mothers in the Southern Health-Board area fell into this category. Classes were considered to be too far away by one third in the Mid-West, a factor which was also identified by 29 per cent of mothers in the West. The highest estimate of 21 per cent for previous attendance at antenatal classes was found for the East, with 19 per cent of mothers in this health-board area, together with the North-East and the South East, believing that the classes were not of any use.

Antenatal Care

The source of antenatal care services prior to the birth of the last baby was found to vary significantly with age, medical-card status, educational experience, employment status, geographical location and social class. Table 6.6 shows that, on average, over half the women attended the public hospital clinic, though this estimate increased to over 60 per cent for mothers under 35 years. While the private clinic/doctor's rooms were attended by more than one in every four mothers, this increased to one in every three for those in the 35–39 age group. For women having their first baby, similar levels of attendance are recorded, with estimates of 61 per cent for those attending the public hospital clinic and 23 per cent for attendances at the private clinic/rooms. There are clear differences in experience according to medical-card status with one out of every three non-medical-card holders attending the private clinic/rooms and three out of every four medical-card holders attending the public hospital clinic.

The relationship between the source of antenatal care and educational experience is evident in Table 6.7. With increasing

levels of education, attendance at the public hospital decreases
from a high of 74 per cent for primary-school leavers to a low of 21
per cent for those with university qualifications. Not surprisingly,
the trend goes in the opposite direction for attendance at private
clinic/rooms with an increase from 10 per cent for mothers with

**Table 6.6: Source of Antenatal Care, by Age Group, Parity,
and Medical-Card Status[†]**

	Source of Antenatal Care			
	Public Hospital Clinic	Semi-Private Clinic	Private Clinic/Rooms	Other
Age Group*	%	%	%	%
18–24	88.2	4.7	3.3	3.9
25–29	75.4	6.6	13.6	4.5
30–34	61.0	8.4	26.8	3.8
35–39	51.7	11.0	32.4	5.0
40–44	54.3	11.4	28.6	5.8
45–49	54.7	8.0	29.3	8.0
50–54	50.8	10.1	27.5	11.7
55–60	49.3	8.3	27.3	15.1
All	57.2	9.1	26.4	7.3
Women Having First Baby**	61.3	9.5	22.9	6.4
Medical-Card Status*				
Yes	78.7	5.1	7.1	9.1
No	46.4	11.5	35.8	6.3
All	57.9	9.0	25.1	7.1

*   p < 0.001.
** p < 0.05.
†   Analysis by age group based on 1,939 (65.1 per cent) women in the sample who have had a baby.
   Analysis by parity based on 276 (14.3 per cent) women who have had only one baby.
   Analysis by medical-card status based on 1,898 (65.7 per cent) women in the sample who have had a baby and for whom medical-card status is known.

Table 6.7: Source of Antenatal Care, by Education Level, and Employment Status[†]

| | Source of Antenatal Care | | | |
	Public Hospital Clinic	Semi-Private Clinic	Private Clinic / Rooms	Other
*Education Level**	%	%	%	%
Primary Cert/Lower	74.0	5.9	9.6	10.5
Inter/Group/Junior Cert	68.3	8.5	17.6	5.6
Leaving Cert/Matric	40.1	12.7	40.5	6.7
Qualification from RTC, etc.	36.2	12.5	48.6	2.7
University Qualification	21.2	6.6	65.5	6.7
All	57.2	9.1	26.4	7.3
*Employment Status**				
Working Full-time	46.2	7.6	39.7	6.5
Working Part-time	56.6	10.8	26.5	6.1
Unemployed	76.4	6.7	11.1	5.9
Home Duties	60.1	9.5	22.8	7.7
Student/Retired/Ill/ Disabled	41.6	13.0	37.8	7.6
All	57.2	9.1	26.4	7.3

* $p < 0.001$.

†   Analysis by education level based on 1,922 (64.5 per cent) women in the sample who have had a baby and for whom education level attained is available.

Analysis by employment status based on 1,939 (65.1 per cent) women in the sample who have had a baby.

primary-level education to 66 per cent for university graduates. Working mothers are the most likely group to attend the private clinic/rooms though over half attend the public hospital clinic. The highest estimate of attendance of 76 per cent found for the public hospital clinic relates to unemployed mothers.

Table 6.8 shows that the geographical differences in the source of antenatal care do not breakdown simply into an urban/rural divide. While over 60 per cent of mothers in the East and the Midlands attend the public hospital clinic, this drops to a

Table 6.8: Source of Antenatal Care, by Health-Board Area, Geographical Location and Social Class[†]

	Source of Antenatal Care			
	Public Hospital Clinic	Semi-Private Clinic	Private Clinic/Rooms	Other
Health-Board Area*	%	%	%	%
East	60.7	17.6	18.3	3.5
Midlands	62.4	6.6	24.2	6.8
Mid-West	51.4	1.9	45.6	1.1
North-East	57.8	10.4	27.6	4.1
North-West	54.9	4.1	20.5	20.6
South	58.9	4.0	35.6	1.6
South-East	45.8	3.0	21.5	29.7
West	54.2	2.8	34.8	8.2
All	57.2	9.1	26.4	7.3
*Geographical Location**				
Rural	55.8	5.1	29.7	9.3
Urban	58.1	11.8	24.2	5.9
All	57.2	9.1	26.4	7.3
*Social Class**				
Higher Professional	28.2	14.7	54.6	2.5
Lower Professional	34.3	11.7	48.1	5.9
Other Non-manual	54.1	12.5	27.0	6.4
Skilled Manual	75.5	5.7	8.7	10.0
Semi-skilled Manual	79.4	4.0	8.4	8.3
Unskilled Manual	81.6	2.1	8.4	7.8
All	56.9	9.2	26.9	6.9

* $p < 0.001$.
†   Analysis by Health Board and geographical location based on 1,939 (65.1 per cent) women in the sample who have had a baby.
    Analysis by social class based on 1,765 (64.8 per cent) women in the sample who have had a baby and for whom social class is known.

low of 46 per cent in the South East. At 18 per cent, the estimate for attendance at the private clinic/rooms is lowest in the East with the highest level of 46 per cent recorded for the Mid-West. The estimate of attendance at public and private clinics is, however, similar for mothers in both rural and urban areas.

The social class distribution in evidence in Table 6.8 for those attending the public hospital clinic and the private clinic/rooms is interesting as the trends go in the opposite direction. While attendance at the public hospital clinic increases from a low of 28 per cent for those in the higher professional group to a high of 82 per cent for the unskilled manual, the 8 per cent of mothers in this group attending the private clinic/rooms increases to a high of 55 per cent for the higher professional group.

The generally high levels of satisfaction with the antenatal care services in evidence from this study are consistent with the findings of a recent study in an Irish maternity hospital (Bosio et al., 1996). The majority of mothers felt that they had enough privacy during their antenatal visits, that they had enough time with their doctor and that both doctors and nurses showed sufficient interest in their concerns. With regard to the time spent with the doctor, there was some difference according to marital status, as 79 per cent of married women thought that they had enough time with the doctor, compared with 61 per cent of single women.

Whether or not the same doctor was seen at each visit and preferences for same are presented in Table 6.9, by medical-card status, educational experience and employment status. While 47 per cent of medical-card holders saw the same doctor at each visit, 66 per cent of the mothers in this group would have preferred to do so. The 69 per cent of non-medical-card holders who saw the same doctor is much closer to the 72 per cent with this preference. This pattern is again in evidence when educational experience and employment status are taken into account, as a smaller proportion of the unemployed and those with primary education saw the same doctor during the visit, compared with the proportion who would have preferred to do so. For working women and those with university qualifications, there were small differences between preferences and experience.

For the majority of mothers, taking time off from work for antenatal visits/classes was not an issue or did not present a problem. There was some variation in experience, however, with 13 per cent of working mothers and 12 per cent of those with RTC-level education estimated to consider that this was a problem. Close to half

Women and Health Care in Ireland

Table 6.9: Saw the Same Doctor/Midwife at Each Visit, or Would Have Liked to Have Seen the Same Doctor/ Midwife, by Medical-Card Status, Education Level, and Employment Status[†]

	Saw the same doctor/midwife at each visit		Would have liked to have seen the same doctor/midwife at each visit		
	Yes	No	Yes	No	Don't Mind
Medical-Card Status*	%	%	%	%	%
Yes	47.2	52.8	66.5	3.5	30.0
No	68.7	31.3	72.2	6.5	21.3
All	61.5	38.5	69.9	5.1	25.0
Education Level**					
Primary Cert/Lower	50.7	49.3	70.3	3.5	26.2
Inter/Group/Junior Cert	55.1	44.9	69.0	5.1	25.9
Leaving Cert/Matric	72.9	27.2	70.5	5.4	24.1
Qualification from RTC, etc.	71.6	28.5	59.6	30.5	9.9
University Qualification	79.9	20.1	81.8	1.5	16.7
All	61.5	38.5	69.9	5.1	25.0
Employment Status***					
Working Full-time	68.7	31.3	76.6	7.8	15.7
Working Part-time	62.5	37.5	70.3	6.5	23.2
Unemployed	58.5	41.6	76.6	5.6	17.8
Home Duties	59.3	40.7	68.7	4.3	27.0
Student/Retired/Ill/Disabled	67.0	33.0	11.3	0.0	88.7
All	61.5	38.5	69.9	5.1	25.0

*   Medical-card status by "saw the same doctor/midwife at each visit": $p < 0.001$.
     Medical-card status by "would have liked to have seen the same doctor/ midwife at each visit": $p < 0.01$.
** $p < 0.001$.
*** Employment status by "saw the same doctor/midwife at each visit": $p < 0.05$.
     Employment status by "would have liked to have seen the same doctor/ midwife at each visit": $p < 0.001$.
†   Analysis by medical-card status based on 1,898 (65.7 per cent) women in the sample who have had a baby and for whom medical-card status is known.
     Analysis by education level based on 1,922 (64.5 per cent) women in the sample who have had a baby and for whom education level attained is available.
     Analysis by employment status based on 1,939 (65.1 per cent) women in the sample who have had a baby.

of the mothers attended for antenatal care during the morning, with a similar estimate attending during the afternoon. These times were also those put forward by the majority of mothers as being the most convenient for visits. University graduates had the lowest estimate for morning attendances (30 per cent), and highest estimates for afternoon and evening attendances — 54 per cent and 16 per cent respectively. The preferred time of attendance for this group was similar, with a slight decrease in the preference for afternoon attendances to 49 per cent and a larger increase in the preference for evening attendances to 19 per cent. The preference for evening attendances also increased marginally among working women to a level of 11 per cent, compared with the estimate of 9 per cent for current experience. Two-thirds of unemployed women would prefer morning clinics, compared with the estimate of 50 per cent currently attending at this time. Among rural mothers, it is estimated that 6 per cent currently attend evening clinics and 48 per cent attend morning clinics. This group, however, expressed a slight preference for more evening clinics (9 per cent) over morning clinics (43 per cent).

The final issue addressed in the area of antenatal care was whether tests should be available in Irish hospitals to show any abnormality in a baby prior to birth. In general, more than three out of every four mothers believe that such tests should be available. Support for this proposal did not vary significantly by medical-card status, educational experience or employment status. There was some variation by age group, with support for the provision of such tests estimated at the 80 per cent level and above for those aged up to 35. The lowest level of support was estimated at 64 per cent for the 55–60 age group. There was also some variation in opinion by geographical location. Estimates of support in excess of 85 per cent were found for the Midlands and the South East with just two-thirds of the mothers in the West falling within this category. The availability of these tests was supported by an estimated 80 per cent of mothers in urban areas, compared with 72 per cent in rural areas. Over 22 per cent of mothers in the West felt that these tests should not be made available, compared with an estimate of 19 per cent for all mothers in rural areas and just 9 per cent for those in urban areas.

Issues arising with regard to the provision of postnatal care will be addressed in the next section.

Postnatal Care

The majority of mothers (86 per cent) considered that they were adequately prepared when going home from the hospital with their babies. There was some difference by age, with the estimate of 78 per cent for the 18–24 year olds contrasting with that of 88 per cent for those aged 35–39. Experience also varied with marital status, as just 69 per cent of single mothers felt adequately prepared to go home with their babies, compared with 87 per cent of those who were married. For the 14 per cent of mothers who did not feel adequately prepared on leaving the hospital, the majority (38 per cent) would have liked to receive further support from the public health nurse. Family, the midwife and the general practitioner were also mentioned by this group of mothers as people from whom additional support would have been desirable.

Following childbirth, the majority of mothers consider that their partner did not feel neglected and that their relationship either did not change or improved. In the majority of cases, the partner provided the most help and support when the mother returned home with the baby. For younger mothers, single mothers and those with medical cards, there was some variation in the sources of support. Among mothers in the 18–24 group, just 28 per cent received the most support from their partners, while parents were the main source of support for 53 per cent of this group. For half the single mothers, parents were again the main source of support, with just 18 per cent estimated to consider their partner in this role. Close to 46 per cent of mothers with medical cards considered the partner as the principle support, compared with 57 per cent for non-medical-card holders. The partner and the parents were each specified by one-third of unemployed women as providing the most help and support following the baby's arrival.

Close to half of the women who have had a baby are estimated to have suffered from postnatal depression or the "baby blues" at some time. The experience of the "baby blues" predominates with an estimate of 38 per cent for mothers, while 11 per cent are estimated to have suffered from postnatal depression. The reported experience of these problems was not found to vary significantly by marital status, medical-card status, employment status or the number of children born to the mother. Variation by age group was significant, with close to half of the women under 30 estimated to have suffered from the "baby blues". Greater awareness of these conditions may, however, be having an effect on the apparently higher levels of experience of the "baby blues" among the younger age groups. While the estimate for postnatal depression dropped from 14 per cent for those with primary education to 6 per cent for university graduates, the experience of the "baby blues" increased from 37 per cent among the group with primary education to 40 per cent for those with a university education. Depression following childbirth is clearly a difficult problem for a significant number of mothers.

Maternity Leave

The 23 per cent of women who, since 1975, had a baby while in paid employment, contrasts with the 15 per cent of women with primary education in this category and the 31 per cent of university graduates. Overall, 83 per cent took maternity leave, though the 69 per cent of women with medical cards or primary education who did so is below the average and substantially less than the estimate of 87 per cent for non-medical-card holders and those with RTC-level education. Almost one in five women with medical cards gave up work when having the baby, compared with 7 per cent for women without medical cards.

Attitudes to Maternity / Paternity Leave

The majority of women who consider that maternity leave is currently adequate does not vary significantly by demographic or geographical factors. While 58 per cent felt that the maternity leave was adequate, 42 per cent felt that it was inadequate. When all women were questioned about their preferences for maternity leave, 58 per cent would prefer six months with half pay while 14 weeks with full pay was the first preference for 30 per cent.

Approximately 69 per cent of women believe that fathers should get paternity leave. Close to 41 per cent of women specify that paternity leave should extend for in excess of three weeks, while two weeks is considered adequate by 38 per cent. Table 6.10 shows that the proportion of women who believe that fathers should receive paid paternity leave drops from a high of 79 per cent for the 30–34 age group to 51 per cent for women aged 55–60. With an estimate of 63 per cent, women with medical cards are somewhat less supportive of paid paternity leave, with 71 per cent

**Table 6.10: Should Fathers Receive Paternity Leave?
by Age Group and Medical-Card Status**

| | Should Fathers Receive Paid Paternity Leave? | |
| | Yes | No |
Age Group*	%	%
18–24	73.2	26.8
25–29	76.2	23.8
30–34	78.8	21.2
35–39	72.4	27.6
40–44	66.9	33.1
45–49	62.4	37.6
50–54	57.1	42.9
55–60	50.8	49.2
All	68.8	31.2
*Medical-Card Status**		
Yes	63.0	37.0
No	71.3	28.8
All	68.8	31.2

*   p < 0.001.

of non-medical-card holders in support. It is clear from Table 6.11 that the support for paid paternity leave increases with level of education from an estimate of 61 per cent for women with primary education to 80 per cent for university graduates. When assessed by employment status, the estimate of 65 per cent found for women engaged in home duties is the lowest level of support for paid paternity leave, while the highest estimate of 74 per cent is found among working women.

Crèche Facilities in the Workplace

Of those in paid employment, just 5 per cent have crèche facilities available at work and only 3 per cent use these facilities. A high of 82 per cent of women believe that crèche facilities should be provided in the workplace. One in four women considers that crèche

Table 6.11: Should Fathers Receive Paternity Leave? by Education Level, Employment Status and Geographical Location

| | Should Fathers Receive Paid Paternity Leave? | |
| | Yes | No |
*Education Level**	%	%
Primary Cert/Lower	61.4	38.6
Inter/Group/Junior Cert	64.2	35.8
Leaving Cert/Matric	73.1	26.9
Qualification from RTC, etc.	75.5	24.5
University Qualification	79.8	20.2
All	68.9	31.1
*Employment Status**		
Working Full-time	73.9	26.1
Working Part-time	68.2	31.8
Unemployed	67.8	32.2
Home Duties	64.6	35.4
Student/Retired/Ill/Disabled	72.2	27.8
All	68.8	31.2
*Geographical Location**		
Rural	64.7	35.3
Urban	71.4	28.6
All	68.8	31.2

* $p < 0.001$.

facilities should be funded by the employer and the parents, while 17 per cent specify that the state should fund such facilities, with the employer and the parents each identified by 14 per cent and 15 per cent, respectively.

The estimates for the very small minority of women who have crèche facilities available in the workplace and who use these facilities do not vary significantly by demographic or geographical factors. There is, however, some significant variation according to whether or not women feel that these facilities should be made available and how they should be funded. Table 6.12 shows that while a significant majority of women believe that crèche facilities should be available in the workplace, the estimate of support drops slightly in the older age groups. With an estimate of 76 per cent, women in rural areas are somewhat less supportive of the provision of such facilities than are women in urban areas, with 84 per cent in support. The analysis by employment status shown in Table 6.13 presents the somewhat surprising result that with an estimate of 78 per cent, women working full-time are the group with the lowest level of support for crèche facilities in the workplace.

Table 6.12: Should Crèche Facilities be Provided in the Workplace and How Should They be Funded? by Age Group

	Should Crèche Facilities be Provided in Workplace?*		How Should Crèche Facilities in the Workplace be Funded?**							
	Yes	No	By State	By employer	By parents	By State and employer	By State and parents	By employer and parents	By combination of all three	Don't know
Age Group	%	%	%	%	%	%	%	%	%	%
18–24	82.2	17.8	17.7	18.4	13.8	7.8	5.9	23.0	11.5	1.9
25–29	83.0	17.0	16.5	14.3	9.2	11.1	10.6	22.9	12.8	2.6
30–34	86.1	13.9	17.4	11.3	14.0	7.2	8.9	26.4	11.2	3.7
35–39	83.3	16.8	13.8	9.9	14.5	8.4	9.4	24.2	16.0	3.7
40–44	83.2	16.8	16.2	15.7	14.3	7.4	6.1	23.4	13.0	4.0
45–49	79.5	20.5	15.5	14.1	19.5	6.7	5.2	26.1	9.5	3.4
50–54	79.3	20.7	16.5	11.6	21.7	12.6	6.1	17.4	10.3	3.8
55–60	68.6	31.4	19.8	10.1	17.9	7.9	5.9	22.1	10.5	5.8
All	81.2	18.8	16.7	13.7	14.9	8.5	7.4	23.5	12.0	3.4

* $p < 0.001$.
** $p < 0.01$.

With the exception of women aged 50–54, Table 6.12 shows that the joint funding of crèche facilities by employers and parents received the highest level of support from all other age groups. Close to 22 per cent of those in the 50–54 group consider that crèche facilities

Table 6.13: Should Crèche Facilities be Provided in the Workplace and How Should They be Funded? by Employment Status and Geographical Location[†]

	Should Crèche Facilities be Provided in Workplace?		How Should Crèche Facilities in the Workplace be Funded?							
	Yes	No	By State	By employer	By parents	By State and employer	By State and parents	By employer and parents	By combination of all three	Don't know
Employment Status*	%	%	%	%	%	%	%	%	%	%
Working Full-time	77.9	22.1	12.4	11.9	17.7	7.9	8.6	24.3	13.7	3.7
Working Part-time	83.9	16.1	17.3	13.2	15.2	7.5	6.6	25.0	13.6	1.6
Unemployed	84.9	15.1	17.8	20.4	9.4	11.4	10.5	13.9	15.2	1.5
Home Duties	82.1	17.9	19.1	13.6	14.7	8.5	6.5	23.5	10.4	3.8
Student/ Retired, Ill/Disabled	85.4	14.6	18.3	17.4	8.5	9.8	6.6	24.9	12.1	2.5
All	81.2	18.8	16.7	13.7	14.9	8.5	7.4	23.5	12.0	3.4
Geographical Location**										
Rural	76.2	23.8	17.4	14.4	18.9	8.2	7.3	17.6	11.2	5.1
Urban	84.4	15.6	16.2	13.3	12.5	8.7	7.5	26.9	12.5	2.4
All	81.2	18.8	16.7	13.7	14.9	8.5	7.4	23.5	12.0	3.4

* $p < 0.01$.

** Geographical Location by "Should Crèche Facilities be Provided?": $p < 0.001$. Geographical Location by "How Should They be Funded?": $p < 0.01$.

†   Analysis based on 2,427 (81.2 per cent) women who think crèche facilities should be provided.

should be funded by parents. For 24 per cent of medical-card holders and 20 per cent of women with primary education, workplace crèches should be funded by the State. Joint funding by employers and parents is the option favoured by about one in four working women, those with university education and those without medical cards. Table 6.13 shows that, with an estimate of 20 per cent, unemployed women favour workplace crèche facilities being funded by the employer.

Family Size

For women aged between 18 and 60, the ideal number of children in a family is estimated to be, on average, 3.1, while the actual/complete family size is estimated to be around three children. When asked about the number of children that they would realistically expect to have in their completed family, 28 per cent said two children, 26 per cent said three children, with four children specified by 17 per cent. While there is some variation between the ideal and the actual family size, the reasons identified for the difference included contraception failure (13 per cent), the fact that it was not possible to have any more children (9 per cent), any more children could not be afforded (9 per cent) and contraception was not used (8 per cent).

Ideal/Actual Family Size

In Table 6.14, the ideal family size relative to the actual/completed family size is shown for each age group and by medical-card status. The mean of the family size that is considered ideal varies from 2.8 for the 30–34 age group to 3.5 for women aged between 50 and 60 years. The mean of the actual/completed family size ranges from 2.6 for those in the 30–34 group to 3.5 for women aged 50–54. For women aged 18–39, the ideal family size is slightly larger than the actual/completed family, while for those aged 40–49, actual/completed family size equals that which is considered ideal. The proportion of women in each age group for whom the ideal equals the actual/completed family size is also presented in Table 6.14. There is a clear age effect in evidence here, with the proportion of women for whom ideal equals actual/completed family size decreasing as age increases. For over 80 per cent of women aged 18–29, ideal equals actual family size, while this is true for less than half the women aged over 50.

Table 6.14: Ideal and Actual/Completed Family Size, Estimated by Age Group and Medical-Card Status

| | *Family Size: Mean Number of Children* | | |
| | *Ideal* | *Actual / Completed* | *Proportion for Whom Ideal = Actual / Completed* |
Age Group			*%*
18–24	3.1	2.8	81.7
25–29	2.9	2.8	80.2
30–34	2.8	2.6	74.4
35–39	3.0	2.9	64.7
40–44	3.3	3.3	56.6
45–49	3.2	3.2	51.1
50–54	3.5	3.5	47.9
55–60	3.5	3.3	41.2
All	3.1	3.0	65.0
Medical-Card Status			
Yes	3.2	3.2	57.3
No	3.1	2.9	68.4
All	3.1	3.0	65.0

For women with medical cards, the ideal family size equals actual/completed family size, while for those without medical cards the ideal is slightly higher when compared with the actual/completed family. Between women with and without medical cards, the difference in the family size considered ideal is considerably smaller than the difference between these two groups in the actual/completed family size.

The mean for ideal and actual/completed family size is shown in Table 6.15 for different levels of educational experience, employment status and geographical location. The estimate for the mean family size which is considered ideal ranges from 3 for women with Leaving Certificate or third-level education to 3.3 for women with primary education. While the estimate for actual/completed family size slightly exceeds that which is considered ideal for women with primary education, for women at all other levels of education the ideal family size is either equal to or slightly larger than the actual/completed family. The actual/completed family size is estimated at 2.7 for women with third-level education compared with 3.4 for women with primary education. While ideal equals actual family size for just 53 per cent of women with primary-level education only, the estimate is closer to 70 per cent for those with Leaving Certificate or third-level qualifications.

Table 6.15: Ideal and Actual/Completed Family Size, Estimated by Education Level, Employment Status and Geographical Location

	Family Size: Mean Number of Children		
	Ideal	*Actual / Completed*	*Proportion for Whom Ideal = Actual / Completed*
Education Level			%
Primary Cert/Lower	3.3	3.4	52.7
Inter/Group/Junior Cert	3.1	3.1	62.8
Leaving Cert/Matric	3.0	2.8	72.2
Qualification from RTC, etc.	3.0	2.7	71.3
University Qualification	3.1	2.7	68.9
All	3.1	3.0	65.0
Employment Status			
Working Full-time	2.9	2.5	71.5
Working Part-time	3.0	3.0	63.5
Unemployed	3.0	2.6	65.5
Home Duties	3.2	3.4	58.9
Student/Retired/Ill/Disabled	3.2	2.8	76.5
All	3.1	3.0	65.0
Geographical Location			
Rural	3.2	3.1	64.6
Urban	3.1	2.9	65.3
All	3.1	3.0	65.0

For working women and unemployed women, the ideal family size is estimated to be around 3 children. This increases to 3.2 for women engaged in home duties. While this latter group of women exceeds the ideal with an estimate of 3.4 for actual/completed family size, the estimate for the ideal family size is either equal to or greater than the actual/completed family for women at all other levels of employment status. Irrespective of geographical location, the ideal family size exceeds the size of the actual/completed family. While women in rural areas consider that 3.2 children is the ideal family size, this contrasts with the 3 children estimated for women in urban areas. At 59 per cent, the proportion of women for whom ideal equals actual/completed family size is smallest for those engaged in home duties.

Parenting Skills

Just over one in every two mothers would have liked to have had more preparation for parenting, compared with 43 per cent who felt that this was not necessary. For close to one in four mothers there had been competition/jealousy between siblings with the arrival of a new baby. Over half the mothers faced with this problem responded by giving the other children extra attention and love, with an additional 30 per cent choosing to involve the other children in helping with the new baby.

Sleeping Position for Baby

Over 70 per cent of mothers correctly recognised that the safest position for a sleeping baby was on the baby's side. The back and the stomach were the positions incorrectly identified by 21 per cent and 9 per cent, respectively. Table 6.16 shows that over two-thirds of the mothers in all age groups correctly reported that the safest sleeping position is on the baby's side, while a high of 28 per cent of those aged 18–24 and 35–39 specified the back, with the stomach identified by around 13 per cent in the 45–54 age group. For three out of four mothers with medical cards, the side was considered the safest sleeping position for the baby, compared with an estimate of 68 per cent for non-medical-card holders.

Table 6.17 shows that the proportion of mothers correctly identifying the side as the safest sleeping position for the baby decreases with increasing levels of education. While the correct response is estimated for 75 per cent of mothers with primary education, this drops to 60 per cent for those with third-level qualifications. The

opposite trend is in evidence for the response that babies should
sleep on their back, with an estimate of 16 per cent at the primary
level increasing to 37 per cent for mothers with university qualifications. While the response to this question did not vary significantly by employment status, the variation by urban/rural location
was found to be significant and is shown in Table 6.17. At 24 per
cent, a substantially higher proportion of women in urban areas
identified the back as the safest sleeping position, compared with
16 per cent in rural areas. The fact that the safest sleeping position
for a baby was on its side was correctly reported for 73 per cent of
women in rural areas and 68 per cent of women in urban areas.

**Table 6.16: Safest Sleeping Position for a Baby, by Age
Group and Medical-Card Status[†]**

	Safest Sleeping Position for a Baby		
	On Back	*On Side[††]*	*On Stomach*
Age Group*	%	%	%
18–24	27.7	68.0	4.3
25–29	22.1	71.3	6.6
30–34	19.6	72.8	7.6
35–39	27.3	65.3	7.4
40–44	19.3	69.8	10.9
45–49	19.8	66.8	13.4
50–54	19.3	68.5	12.2
55–60	12.9	78.9	8.2
All	20.6	70.1	9.3
Medical-Card Status**			
Yes	17.3	73.8	8.9
No	22.2	68.0	9.9
All	20.4	70.1	9.5

* $p < 0.01$.
** $p < 0.03$.
†   Analysis by age group based on 1,939 (65.1 per cent) women in the sam-
    ple who have had a baby.
    Analysis by medical-card status based on 1,898 (65.7 per cent) women in
    the sample who have had a baby and for whom medical-card status is
    known.
†† Most appropriate response.

Table 6.17: Safest Sleeping Position for a Baby, by Education Level and Geographical Location[†]

	Safest Sleeping Position for a Baby		
	On Back	On Side[††]	On Stomach
Education Level*	%	%	%
Primary Cert/Lower	15.6	74.6	9.8
Inter/Group/Junior Cert	19.2	70.0	10.8
Leaving Cert/Matric	22.1	69.4	8.5
Qualification from RTC, etc.	30.0	60.1	9.9
University Qualification	36.8	60.0	3.2
All	20.6	70.1	9.3
*Geographical Location**			
Rural	15.5	72.8	11.7
Urban	24.0	68.3	7.7
All	20.6	70.1	9.3

* $p < 0.001$.

† Analysis by education level based on 1,922 (64.5 per cent) women in the sample who have had a baby for whom education level attained is available. Analysis by geographical location based on 1,939 (65.1 per cent) women in the sample who have had a baby.

†† Most appropriate response.

Conclusion

Given the association between attendance at antenatal classes and improvement in birth outcomes, it is of some concern that less than one-third of Irish mothers are estimated to have attended antenatal classes prior to the birth of their last baby. When asked why antenatal classes were not attended, access was found to be a major issue with an estimated 18 per cent reporting that none were available and 17 per cent considering that the classes were too far away. Additional reasons given for non-attendance were that they "didn't think they were of any use" (15 per cent), they had done them before (13 per cent) and they had "no time" (11 per cent). It is interesting that a 1990 study of predictors of attendance at antenatal classes among a sample of women in England found that transport difficulties were the only "practical" reason for non-attendance (Mitchie, Marteau, Kidd, 1990). This study concluded

that women's intentions at 28 weeks pregnancy concerning attendance were the best predictor of subsequent attendance, while non-
attendance was most likely to be associated with single women and
women on low incomes. This finding would seem to be supported
by the findings presented here, as only 2.5 per cent of women re-
ferred to the costliness of classes as a reason for non-attendance.

The Canadian study by Stewart et al. (1990) found that major
categories of deterrents to early prenatal class attendance included
the low level of public knowledge about availability and usefulness,
and low physician–patient referral. The recommendation that
early attendance at antenatal classes should be promoted through
a wide range of outlets in the community would also seem to be
relevant to the Irish context. In addition, the access problem en-
countered by a substantial proportion of Irish women should be
addressed by the service-providers to ensure that women recognising the need for this service can avail of classes locally.

The fact that 42 per cent of women who took maternity leave
from work when having a baby felt that the leave was inadequate
is cause for concern. More than one in every two women considered that six months with half pay would be required for adequate maternity leave. Approximately three times as many
women with medical cards compared with non-medical-card holders gave up work when having a baby. The majority of women believe that paternity leave should be available to all fathers.

While 82 per cent of women believe that crèche facilities
should be provided in the workplace, only 5 per cent of women in
paid employment have crèche facilities available at work. The
preference for more preparation for parenting expressed by the
majority of women should be taken seriously in view of the finding that 30 per cent did not know that the safest position for a
sleeping baby was on its side.

Insufficient attendance at antenatal classes and the desire for
better preparation for parenting may be related, given the conclusion of a recent study that antenatal education may provide an
opportunity "to use the 'teachable moment' of pregnancy to em-
bark on a forward-thinking approach to assisting new parents to
establish solid foundations for their own and their children's future" (Chalmers and McIntyre, 1994).

7

Attitudes and Approaches to Breast-feeding

Introduction

Scientific evidence indicates that breast-feeding has a significant positive effect on the health of the infant, on the health of the mother, and on the mother–child relationship. In addition, breast-feeding is considered to have positive economic benefits as well as being environmentally friendly (Wellstart International, 1993). Specifically, breast-fed infants have been found to have better protection against acute infectious diseases and certain chronic diseases (Department of Health, 1994). Significant advantages in cognitive function have also been associated with breast-feeding of healthy babies (Standing Committee on Nutrition of the British Paediatric Association, 1994).

The incidence of mothers breast-feeding in Ireland has been estimated to be in the region of 30 per cent, which is considered low by international standards (Department of Health, 1994). This contrasts with the United States which experienced a decrease in the proportion of mothers breast-feeding from a high of 60 per cent in the early 1980s to approximately 52 per cent in 1989, though the opposite trend has been in evidence in a number of European countries over the same period (Formon, 1987; Ryan et al., 1991). From an estimate of 51 per cent in 1975, the incidence of breast-feeding in England and Wales increased to 64 per cent in 1990 (Martin and Monk, 1980; White, Freeth and O'Brien, 1990). Norway is reported to be the European country with the highest incidence and duration of breast-feeding, with an estimated 90 per cent of Norwegian women breast-feeding for at least one week (Liestol, Rosenberg and Wallore, 1988; Department of Health, 1994). Since the early 1980s the mean frequency of breast-feeding at three months has been maintained at around the 70 per cent level in Norway (Helsing and Kjaernes, 1985).

A 1991 specification of Department of Health policy recognises that "breast-feeding is the most satisfactory method of infant feeding for the normal infant from birth" and seeks to promote and encourage this approach to infant feeding.[1] Some understanding of the extent to which this policy is reflected in practice among Irish women may be gathered from the information on attitudes to breast-feeding and experiences of breast-feeding reported in this chapter.

From the results of the national survey it is estimated that 59 per cent of mothers never breast-feed. Of those who do, 14 per cent breast-feed their first baby, 12 per cent breast-feed some of their babies and 15 per cent breast-feed all of their babies. Over 70 per cent of mothers who breast-feed do so because it is considered best for the baby, while 9 per cent do so for convenience. This finding supports the results of a number of previous studies where perceived benefits to the health of the infant was found to be one of the strongest influences on the decision to breast-feed (Novotny et al., 1994; Alexy and Martin, 1994; Fitzpatrick, Fitzpatrick and Darling, 1994). Almost half of the women who breast-feed do so for less than six weeks, while a quarter breast-feed for three months. Over 12 per cent of mothers breast-feed for longer than six months. An estimate of 46 per cent consider that a woman cannot take the pill when breast-feeding while 45 per cent do not know whether or not this is advisable.[2]

Altogether, over two-fifths of women stop breast-feeding because the baby is not getting enough or because they feel it is time to stop. In addition, 13 per cent stop because it is too demanding while an additional 11 per cent stop because of breast problems. Close to one in four mothers consider that they were made to feel embarrassed when breast-feeding while 83 per cent believe that facilities in public places are not adequate for breast-feeding. While these estimates relate to women who did breast-feed, previous Irish studies have found that close to 10 per cent of bottle-feeders

---

[1]   Code of practice for the marketing of infant formulae in the Republic of Ireland, 1991.

[2]   It should be noted that while it is safe to take the *mini-pill* while breast-feeding, the combined oral contraceptive pill should not be taken while breast-feeding.

mentioned embarrassment as one of the reasons why they did not breast-feed (Fitzpatrick, Fitzpatrick and Darling, 1994; McSweeney and Kevany, 1982).

Experience of Breast-feeding

In the bivariate analyses, whether or not a mother breast-fed one or more of her babies was found to be significantly related to age, medical-card status, attendance at antenatal classes, educational experience, employment status and social class. In the multivariate analysis, however, medical-card status and employment status were found to be confounded within education and social class. Breast-feeding experience did not vary significantly by geographical location. Table 7.1 shows that over one-fifth of mothers aged between 35 and 44 breast-fed all of their babies. With an estimate of just over 50 per cent, this group also accounted for the lowest proportion of mothers who have never breast-fed. While over 85 per cent of mothers aged 18–24 have never breast-fed, this is followed by an estimate of 68 per cent for mothers in the 45–49 age group.

Interesting information on breast-feeding experience according to whether or not antenatal classes were attended in preparation for the birth of the last baby is presented in Table 7.1. The estimates for breast-feeding of first babies and all babies is higher among mothers who attended antenatal classes than for non-attendees. Of those attending antenatal classes, the 46 per cent who have never breast-fed contrasts with the estimate of 65 per cent for mothers who did not attend classes.

The proportion of mothers breast-feeding is shown in Table 7.2 to be clearly related to educational experience. The higher the level of educational achievement, the greater the proportion of mothers who breast-feed. For women with university qualifications, over one-third have breast-fed all their babies, over one-fifth have breast-fed their first babies and just 28 per cent have never breast-fed. Close to three-quarters of women with primary education only have never breast-fed, while just 5 per cent have breast-fed all of their babies.

The social class relationship with breast-feeding experience is clearly in evidence from Table 7.2. The higher professional group accounts for the highest proportion of mothers who have breast-fed their first baby, some of their babies and all of their babies, and the lowest estimate for those who have never breast-fed any of their babies. Three out of four mothers from the semi-skilled manual and unskilled manual groups have never breast-fed any of their babies, and these groups also account for the lowest proportion of mothers who have breast-fed some or all of their babies.

Table 7.1: Number of Babies Breast-fed, by Age Group, Attendance at Antenatal Classes and Medical-Card Status[†]

	Number of Babies Breast-fed			
	First Baby	*Some of her Babies*	*All of her Babies*	*Never Breast-fed*
Age Group*	*%*	*%*	*%*	*%*
18–24	9.0	3.3	2.5	85.3
25–29	17.7	6.8	9.4	66.1
30–34	16.8	7.0	18.1	58.1
35–39	16.0	12.1	21.6	50.4
40–44	10.2	16.5	21.4	51.9
45–49	7.6	14.8	9.4	68.3
50–54	12.9	15.2	12.9	59.0
55–60	18.2	12.9	9.7	59.2
All	13.8	12.0	15.0	59.2
Attendance at Antenatal Classes*				
Yes	19.5	10.6	23.6	46.3
No	11.2	12.7	11.1	65.0
All	13.8	12.0	15.0	59.2

*   p < 0.001.
†   Analysis based on 1,939 (65.1 per cent) women in the sample who have had a baby.

While the majority of women who breast-feed do so for less that six weeks, between one-fifth and one-quarter continue breast-feeding for up to three months. There is some variation in the duration of breast-feeding by age group, with women in the younger age groups breast-feeding for somewhat shorter periods than those in the older age groups. Between 80 and 90 per cent of women up to the age of 30 breast-feed for less than three months, compared with between 60 per cent and 70 per cent for those aged 35–44. Between 15 per cent and 20 per cent of women in this older age group breast-feed for longer than six months, compared with around 10 per cent in the younger age group.

Table 7.2: Number of Babies Breast-fed, by Education Level and Social Class[†]

	Number of Babies Breast-fed			
	First Baby	*Some of her Babies*	*All of her Babies*	*Never Breast-fed*
Education Level*	%	%	%	%
Primary Cert/Lower	9.3	13.1	5.1	72.5
Inter/Group/Junior Cert	13.6	11.8	11.0	63.6
Leaving Cert/Matric	15.4	10.4	23.3	50.9
Qualification from RTC, etc.	21.8	20.1	22.0	36.2
University Qualification	22.2	13.4	36.6	27.8
All	13.7	12.1	15.1	59.1
Social Class*				
Higher Professional	17.9	16.7	33.8	31.7
Lower Professional	14.4	14.0	25.7	45.9
Other Non-Manual	16.6	10.2	13.5	59.3
Skilled Manual	10.9	14.8	7.0	67.3
Semi-skilled Manual	12.5	7.6	4.7	75.2
Unskilled manual	6.4	10.5	8.9	74.2
All	13.9	12.2	15.3	58.7

* $p < 0.001$.

†   Analysis by education level based on 1,922 (64.5 per cent) women in the sample who have had a baby and for whom education level attained is available.

Analysis by social class based on 1,765 (64.8 per cent) women in the sample who have had a baby and for whom social class is known.

Unemployed women were also more likely to breast-feed longer, with 51 per cent estimated to breast-feed for longer than six months. The variation in the length of time spent breast-feeding, by educational experience, is interesting, with close to half of the group between primary and RTC-level education breast-feeding for up to six weeks, compared with over one-third for women with university education. Over one-fifth of this latter group of women breast-feed for longer than six months, compared with just over 5 per cent for women with primary education only.

Following these bivariate analyses, multivariate analyses of breast-feeding behaviour were undertaken. Logistic regression models were estimated for mothers who had only one child and for mothers who had more than one child. The logistic regression analysis of whether or not mothers with one child had breast-fed found that attendance at antenatal classes and level of education had significant effects. Mothers of single children who had attended antenatal classes and those with higher levels of education were more likely to breast-feed.

The logistic regression analysis of breast-feeding behaviour for mothers with more then one child found that age, education level, social class, number of children and attendance at antenatal classes prior to the birth of the last baby were significantly related to outcome. The model provided a good fit of the data and the parameter estimates are presented in Table A8, Appendix 3. These results show that mothers who attend antenatal classes are more likely to breast-feed, whereas those who don't are more likely not to. The probability of breast-feeding increases with age, education level and the number of children. Mothers in the higher social classes, with more than one child, are also more likely to breast-feed.

The results of the multivariate analysis presented here are consistent with those produced by previous studies both in Ireland and elsewhere. The Fitzpatrick, Fitzpatrick and Darling (1994) study of Irish women found that the decision to breast-feed was influenced by age, social class, level of education and the additional factors of marital status and whether or not a semiprivate or private clinic was attended. Age and education were found to be significant predictors of breast-feeding behaviour in a study of Danish women by Fleischer et al. (1994), and education and attendance at antenatal classes were found to be significant factors in studies of breast-feeding among English women (Bruce et al., 1991; Salt et al., 1994).

The combined effect of the significant independent variables for the multivariate analysis of breast-feeding behaviour for mothers with more than one child is effectively illustrated by the examples of predicted probabilities presented in Table 7.3. This table shows that 89 per cent of mothers aged 25–29, with two children, with primary education and a semi-skilled manual background, who did not attend antenatal classes would be expected never to breast-feed. This estimate drops to 18 per cent for higher professional mothers aged 30–34, with three children, with a university education, who attended antenatal classes.

Table 7.3: Estimated Percentages of Mothers who Breast-fed for Specified Characteristics Defined According to Age, Education, Social Class and Attendance at Antenatal Classes

	Mothers	*First Baby* %	*Some Babies* %	*All Babies* %	*Never Breast-fed* %
1	Aged 25–29 Primary-level education Semi-skilled manual Two children Did not attend antenatal classes	3	5	2	89
2	Aged 40–44 Leaving Cert education Lower professional Four children Attended antenatal classes	7	15	53	25
3	Aged 30–34 University-level education Higher professional Three children Attended antenatal classes	10	14	58	18

Termination of Breast-feeding

A wide range of reasons as to why mothers stop breast-feeding have been put forward, with some variation in evidence by age, medical-card status, educational experience and employment status. Social class differences in the reasons for stopping breast-feeding were not significant. The reasons cited by the different age groups and by medical-card status are presented in Table 7.4.

Table 7.4: Reasons for Stopping Breast-Feeding, by Age Group and Medical-Card Status[†]

	\multicolumn{11}{c}{*Reasons for Stopping Breast-Feeding*}										
	Went back to work	*Diffi-culty in Social Situ-ations*	*Dis-liked it*	*Too demand-ing*	*Baby not sett-ling*	*Baby not getting enough*	*Baby got teeth*	*Baby old enough to drink from cup*	*Felt it was time to stop*	*Breast prob-lems*	*Other*
Age Group*	%	%	%	%	%	%	%	%	%	%	%
18–24	4.5	0.0	0.0	3.6	0.0	16.6	0.0	0.0	22.5	42.5	10.4
25–29	25.9	3.4	5.6	9.7	0.0	22.6	0.0	0.7	8.0	11.4	12.9
30–34	15.2	1.4	2.5	10.7	3.1	18.9	0.0	5.6	14.6	10.4	17.7
35–39	9.5	0.0	3.5	11.7	2.6	18.1	0.5	6.3	23.2	10.3	14.1
40–44	7.4	2.6	3.3	14.7	1.3	19.8	1.0	5.8	25.9	10.6	7.5
45–49	2.6	0.0	1.6	9.9	6.3	21.9	1.0	3.2	24.5	18.9	10.1
50–54	1.8	1.8	3.6	16.3	8.1	25.1	0.9	3.3	17.3	10.3	11.5
55–60	3.1	0.6	2.4	13.7	4.9	31.5	3.4	6.9	20.8	6.2	6.5
All	8.7	1.3	3.1	12.5	3.5	21.8	0.9	5.0	20.3	11.3	11.6
MCS **											
Yes	2.4	0.5	4.2	11.6	2.9	25.0	1.9	6.3	18.4	11.9	15.0
No	11.0	1.5	2.8	12.1	3.9	21.1	0.6	4.5	20.9	11.0	10.6
All	8.7	1.2	3.2	12.0	3.6	22.2	1.0	5.0	20.2	11.2	11.8

* $p < 0.001$.

** $p < 0.01$.

†   Analysis by age group based on 794 (40.8 per cent) mothers who had breast-fed a baby.

Analysis by medical-card status based on 767 (40.4 per cent) mothers who had breast-fed a baby and for whom medical-card status is known.

Note: MCS = Medical-Card Status.

A high estimate of 43 per cent of women in the 18–24 group ter-
minated because of breast problems, compared with an average of
11 per cent for all women. For the same age group, 23 per cent felt
that it was time to stop and 17 per cent stopped when they felt
that the baby was not getting enough. It is not particularly surprising that for close to one in five women in the 25–29 age group
returning to work is the important reason for finishing breast-
feeding. The fact that the baby is not getting enough and that the
women feel that it is time to stop are among the most common
reasons put forward across all age groups. The greatest difference
between those with and without medical cards is found for stopping breast-feeding because of the need to return to work. While
11 per cent of non-medical-card holders had to stop breast-feeding
because of a return to work, this contrasts with an estimate of 2
per cent for mothers with medical cards.

The reasons presented for stopping breast-feeding are presented by different levels of educational experience and employment status in Table 7.5. While the high frequency factors continue to be the same as those mentioned above, it is noteworthy
that 23 per cent of mothers with university qualifications had to
stop breast-feeding because of a return to work. The 15 per cent of
mothers with primary education only who stopped because they
felt that the baby was too demanding contrasts with the estimate
of 6 per cent for mothers with university education. The fact that
the baby was not getting enough is the reason for the high of 33
per cent of mothers with RTC qualifications.

Table 7.5 shows that over one-quarter of working women had
to terminate because of a return to work, which might not be surprising, though the 21 per cent of mothers engaged in home duties
who felt that it was too demanding is somewhat higher than expected. Feeling that it is time to stop is the reason for an estimated 62 per cent of unemployed mothers. When asked whether
anything would have helped them to continue breast-feeding,
close to two thirds of women said that nothing would have en-
abled them to continue. More than 10 per cent of mothers feel
however, that more help from the nurse or health visitor would be
of assistance in continuing breast-feeding. While information and
support from health professionals for breast-feeding has been
found to be positively associated with the decision to breast-feed,
the absence of this assistance has been found to be a source of
discontent for breast-feeding mothers (Rajan, 1993).

Table 7.5: Reasons for Stopping Breast-Feeding, by Education Level and Employment Status[†]

	Reasons for Stopping Breast-Feeding										
	Went back to work	Diffi-culty in Social Situ-ations	Dis-liked it	Too demand-ing	Baby not sett-ling	Baby not getting en-ough	Baby got teeth	Baby old enough to drink from cup	Felt it was time to stop	Breast prob-lems	Other
*Education Level**	%	%	%	%	%	%	%	%	%	%	%
Primary Cert/ Lower	2.5	1.5	3.9	14.6	5.3	29.2	1.3	2.8	16.7	11.8	10.3
Inter/ Group/ Junior Cert	5.2	1.8	5.8	13.6	3.4	21.8	2.2	4.4	17.3	12.0	12.7
Leaving Cert/ Matric	10.5	0.9	1.5	12.8	3.5	18.6	0.3	6.6	24.5	10.8	10.0
Qual. from RTC, etc.	9.5	2.4	2.1	8.6	3.2	32.8	0.0	2.4	11.1	10.5	17.5
University Qual.	22.5	0.0	1.0	6.4	1.0	15.7	0.0	6.0	23.7	9.3	14.5
All	8.7	1.3	3.1	12.5	3.5	21.8	0.9	5.0	20.3	11.3	11.6
*Employ-ment Status**											
Working Full-time	25.9	0.9	0.4	11.8	2.6	18.4	0.0	3.1	15.2	11.0	10.6
Working Part-time	8.6	3.5	3.4	12.3	5.1	16.6	0.5	5.4	26.5	10.3	7.8
Un-employed	0.0	0.0	0.0	0.0	3.9	14.6	0.0	14.1	62.3	5.0	0.0
Home Duties	1.6	1.2	4.4	13.0	3.8	24.5	1.3	5.4	20.6	11.4	13.0
Student/ Retired/ Ill/Disabled	15.6	0.0	0.0	16.7	0.0	0.0	10.0	10.0	23.9	23.9	0.0
All	8.7	1.3	3.1	12.5	3.5	21.8	0.9	5.0	20.3	11.3	11.6

* $p < 0.001$.

†   Analysis by education level based on 786 (40.9 per cent) mothers who had breast-fed a baby and for whom education level attained is available. Analysis by employment status based on 794 (40.8 per cent) mothers who had breast-fed a baby.

Breast-Feeding in Public

On average, three out of four mothers said that they had never been made to feel embarrassed while breast-feeding. A high of 83 per cent of mothers however, feel that facilities in public places are not adequate for breast-feeding, compared with the estimate of 8 per cent who feel that public facilities are adequate. These estimates do not differ significantly according to medical-card status, educational experience, employment status, geographical location or social class. It is noteworthy that the proportion of women in the 25–39 age group who feel that public facilities are inadequate is closer to 90 per cent, with an estimate of 96 per cent recorded for women aged 18–24.

Conclusion

It is clear from the study results presented here that breast-feeding continues to be the option of choice for a minority of Irish women. While the promotion of breast-feeding has long been a policy of the Department of Health, the continuing low rates prompted the Minister for Health in 1992 to appoint a National Committee to Promote Breast-feeding. This committee was charged with responsibility for developing a national policy to promote breast-feeding in Ireland. This policy was published in 1994 (Department of Health, 1994).

The general objectives for the national policy on breast-feeding include:

- Increasing the percentage of mothers who initiate breast-feeding

- Increasing the percentage who practise exclusive breast-feeding to at least four months and thereafter with appropriate weaning foods.

In order to achieve these objectives, the strategies proposed by the committee include the development and active implementation of breast-feeding policies in maternity hospitals and units and at the community-care level, in addition to providing the necessary educational support at the training level.

While the policy-makers have accepted the principle that where breast-feeding is a feasible option, it is the best option for infant health, the study results presented here would suggest that this is still not generally accepted among mothers faced with the choice of breast-feeding or bottle-feeding. The finding that breast-feeding continues to be the choice of the better-educated and professional woman highlights the need to find more effective channels for imparting information on the benefits of breast-feeding to all women, and particularly to expectant and new mothers. This factor has been highlighted in a number of other studies where education about breast-feeding at an early age has been found to have a positive influence when faced with the decision to breast-feed (Fitzpatrick, Fitzpatrick and Darling, 1994; Quarles et al., 1994; Rajan, 1993). The fact that attendance at antenatal classes has also been found to be positively associated with breast-feeding behaviour provides further support for the recommendation in the previous chapter that higher levels of attendance at antenatal classes should be actively pursued.

In addition to the influence of education and social class, the cultural influence on choice of feeding options is strong. In this regard, the authors of a study of breast-feeding in two English districts concluded that "health education is unlikely to change breast-feeding practices unless prevailing cultural attitudes also change" (Salt et al., 1994: 291).

An increase in the proportion of Irish mothers who choose to breast-feed would therefore seem to warrant a multi-faceted approach. To some extent, this is reflected in the 1994 report of the National Committee to Promote Breast-feeding where the promotion of breast-feeding in the wider community is recognised as an important objective. It would seem, however, that if it is to be successful, the implementation of this objective will require a strong proactive approach on the part of health professionals, health educators and all involved with the provision of services to expectant and new mothers.

8

Conclusions and
Recommendations

Introduction

The national survey of women's health needs initiated by the National Maternity Hospital, Holles Street, Dublin, to commemorate its centenary represents the first national study of Irish women's understanding of their own health needs and their attitudes to many different types of behaviour, including smoking, alcohol consumption, fertility control, breast-feeding etc. An important objective for the commissioning of this survey was the provision of a more informed platform for decision-making and policy development in regard to support and service provision for the protection, maintenance and improvement of the health of women in Ireland. As the survey involved the completion of a questionnaire with 139 questions for close to 3,000 women nationally, a very large data base on a wide range of important issues has been assembled. The subject areas covered included nutrition, sex education, sexually transmitted diseases, family planning, maternity leave, hospital services for mothers, breast-feeding, parenting skills, gynaecology, family size and lifestyles.

Given the size of the data base, it has been necessary to be selective about the information presented in this book. In deciding on the areas for analysis, we have concentrated on those issues which are very directly related to women's health and their interface with the health services. Given the objective of facilitating more informed policy-making in regard to the provision of services concerned with women's health, there is a strong emphasis on the socio-demographic perspective in the completed analysis. The potential relevance of these findings may be more fully appreciated when considered against the background of the objectives for government policy on women's health services proposed in the Department of Health's 1994 strategy document, *Shaping a Healthier Future*, and the 1995 discussion document, *Developing a Policy for Women's Health*. These objectives include the following:

- To ensure that women's health needs are identified and planned for in a comprehensive way.

- To ensure that women receive the health and welfare services that they need at the right time and in a way that respects their dignity and individuality. They must have ease of access to, and continuity of, care.

- To promote greater consultation with women about their health and welfare needs. This must be done at national, regional and local level.

- To promote within the health services a greater participation by women, both in the more senior positions and at the representative level (Department of Health, 1994b: 55).

While all of the areas considered here yield important findings for consideration in pursuit of the policy objectives for women's health studies, a number of general conclusions emerging from the initial review of results require specific attention. The first is cause for concern as this survey highlights serious and pervasive gaps in the basic information available to many women concerning the maintenance and advancement of good physical, mental and reproductive health. What is particularly worrying is the fact that these information gaps may be most prevalent amongst women at greatest risk of disadvantage, including those with less education and without employment. The evidence that is now available clearly points to the need to ensure that the development and implementation of all future policies concerned with women's health have specific regard to the needs of disadvantaged women at greatest risk of ill health. It is readily recognised that targeting certain risk factors to encourage behaviour with more positive health benefits may be an incomplete response to the deeply disadvantaged context in which too many women exist (Link and Phelan, 1995). A recognition of the relatively greater needs of these women would, however, be an important first step in gaining priority status for disadvantaged women on the policy-makers agenda and would be consistent with the active pursuit of the objective of equity in the health-care system, as proposed in the national health strategy, *Shaping Healthier Future* (Department of Health, 1994b).

On the positive side, the findings presented here indicate that Irish women may be more open and progressive than has traditionally been assumed to be the case. For the first time, Irish women nationally have been asked for their opinion on such issues as where condoms should be on sale, whether sterilisation and genetic screening services should be available in public hospitals, etc. In responding to these questions, the majority of women have indicated an openness and a tolerance which in many instances may be an advancement on the assumptions that have traditionally informed public policy on these issues. This survey has shown that Irish women generally have informed, independent opinions on issues of importance to their welfare and that of the society at large — factors which must undoubtedly be taken into consideration when policy-makers and politicians approach the development of future policy in these areas and the implementation of the health strategy objectives proposed by the Department of Health (Department of Health, 1994b, 1995a). Some of the main findings from this study, together with the recommended policy response will now be summarised.

Substance Use and Abuse

Despite the risks to their own health and to that of their unborn babies, 29 per cent of Irish women smoke regularly, 45 per cent of mothers who smoke continued to smoke while pregnant and one in every five women smokers say that they would smoke during a future pregnancy. While alcohol consumption during pregnancy is also associated with adverse birth outcomes, only 45 per cent of Irish women say that they would give up drinking during a future pregnancy. Tranquilliser use to cope with stress is significantly higher for women with medical cards than for other women.

Recommendations

If smoking and alcohol misuse by women in general, and pregnant women in particular, is to be reduced, strategic information and intervention programmes will need to be actively implemented in the Irish context. These programmes could include mass media campaigns highlighting the risks of smoking and alcohol consumption during pregnancy and smoking cessation programmes designed specifically to motivate pregnant women to stop smoking.

Professional training of physicians, nurses and other health professionals and their systematic intervention in programmes intended to stop smoking and alcohol misuse would be expected to facilitate the promotion of healthier lifestyles for all women, and pregnant women in particular.

The development and implementation of the comprehensive strategies necessary to stop smoking and alcohol misuse by women will need to be based on the essential components of research, outreach, education and advocacy.

Sex Education

The fact that formal sex education has become more accessible to Irish women is indicated by the finding that the younger age cohorts report positively that sex education has been received. Despite this development, one in four women did not know at what stage of the menstrual cycle they are most likely to become pregnant, and this estimate rises to 40 per cent for unemployed women. The level of awareness of the population groups most at risk of the AIDS virus and the most effective means of avoiding exposure to AIDS have been found to vary according to level of education, employment status and medical-card status. These findings indicate that the effectiveness of the strategies thus far devised to convey this information to the population at large may not be consistent for all women.

Recommendations

It is essential to ensure that sex education programmes aimed at post-pubescent girls specifically address all issues arising with regard to the risk of becoming pregnant.

Ensuring that all sexually-active women are fully informed about the risk factors associated with infection by the AIDS virus and how these risks can be avoided must now be recognised as a public health priority. Given the finding that the knowledge gaps on this question vary according to level of education and employment status, there would seem to be good grounds for targeting programmes at those population groups where current levels of information are considered least adequate.

Family Planning

While two-thirds of Irish women are sexually active, only half consider that family planning advice is easily accessible in their area. More rural women than urban women consider that family planning services are not adequately accessible to them, with the perceived adequacy of this information reported to be lowest for unemployed women, students, and those who are ill or disabled. While the general practitioner tends to be the source of family planning information for more rural women, and the family planning clinic is more often used by urban women, as many as one in four women in certain geographical areas would not seek family planning advice locally. The 43 per cent of sexually-active women with only a primary education and not using any method of family planning contrasts with the estimate of 23 per cent for women with a university education. Single women and married women have significantly different preferences for the method of family planning used. Almost 40 per cent of single women choose the combined pill and 31 per cent use condoms compared with estimates of 12 per cent and 21 per cent, respectively for the proportion of married women using the same methods. More than four out of every five Irish women believe that condoms should be sold in Ireland without a prescription and that sterilisation should be available to women and men in all publicly funded Irish hospitals.

Recommendations

Support for a concerted strategy aimed at the immediate implementation of the family planning guidelines issued to health boards by the Minister for Health is clearly indicated. This strategy must be concerned with ensuring that family planning services are available to all women in need of these services, irrespective of where they live and their financial and social circumstances. Plans for the improvement in the availability of family planning services should also take account of the fact that the most frequently used sources of information on these services are, in order of importance: the general practitioner, the family planning clinic and the health centre.

The fact that condoms are now available in Ireland without a prescription is supported by the majority of Irish women. It should also be recognised that the majority of women believe that condoms should be available in chemists, supermarkets, pubs, discos and any retail outlet that wants to stock them.

The availability of sterilisation services for women and men in all publicly funded hospitals is clearly supported by the majority of Irish women.

Gynaecology

Like other body systems, the female reproductive system requires particular care and maintenance if it is to remain healthy. The hormonal changes that are associated with this system mean that women may need to take specific initiatives at different stages of the life cycle to maintain good health. It is therefore all the more cause for concern that the survey questions concerned with gynaecological issues revealed some of the most pervasive gaps in the prevailing knowledge about the initiatives that women need to take to maintain a good healthy functioning reproductive system for as long as possible. While it is recommended that all women should have a cervical smear test every 2 or 3 years, one in four women reports that it is over three years since she had her last smear test. Given the recommendation that all women should conduct routine self-examination of their breasts, it is of considerable concern that 39 per cent of women say that they never undertake such examinations. The fact that one-quarter of these women do not know how to conduct such examinations or are afraid of what they would find is indicative of an information gap that could have serious consequences for the health of these women.

Overall, one in five women considers that she does not have enough information on the menopause, and this estimate increases to one in four for unemployed women. While the use of hormone replacement therapy (HRT) to alleviate symptoms of the menopause is relatively recent, one in four women does not know why it might be prescribed, an estimate that increases to one in three for medical-card holders and 42 per cent for unemployed women. A similar pattern emerged when questions about osteoporosis were raised, with an overall estimate that one in four women does not understand this condition and one in three unemployed women and those with only a primary-level education does not know the cause of this condition or how it could be avoided. These results show very clearly that too many women do not have the basic information necessary for the protection of their own health, such as when to have a smear test, when and how to conduct breast self-examination and how to avoid osteoporosis.

Recommendations

The information gaps identified here should be very directly addressed when developing and implementing health-promotion policies for women. Basic information on when, and under what circumstances, women should have cervical smear tests, and when and how to conduct breast self-examination should be considered essential for all women. Those authorities with responsibility for health promotion at the health-board and national level should therefore be using all possible information channels to get this essential information across to post-pubescent girls and women. Targeted strategies will again be necessary to reach the more disadvantaged women who tend to fall through the gaps in the traditional approaches to health promotion and information dissemination. In addition, the recommendation by the *Report of the Second Commission on the Status of Women* (1993) that cervical smear tests should be made available for screening as well as diagnostic purposes under the General Medical Services scheme should be implemented as a matter of urgency.

Strategies to inform women about the menopause, and how associated symptoms may be avoided or moderated, must also be recognised as an important element of health promotion policy for women. In particular, women in general should be better informed about approaches to minimising the risk factors for osteoporosis. Women who have traditionally been more marginalised and more vulnerable to avoidable morbidity should be specifically targeted by health promotion policies concerned with these conditions.

Having a Baby: Antenatal and Postnatal Experience, Maternity Leave, Family Size and Parenting Skills

When questioned about the services and the circumstances associated with childbirth, three out of four mothers believed that tests should be available in Irish hospitals to show if a baby has any abnormality prior to birth. Given that attendance at antenatal classes has been shown to improve birth outcomes, it is worrying that just 31 per cent of Irish mothers attended these classes in preparation for the birth of their last baby. While this rate of attendance is considered low for this population as a whole, it drops to even lower levels for particular women. One in four rural mothers attended classes, compared with one in three mothers in urban areas. The majority of rural mothers not attending classes reported that they were either too far away or not available. Only 18 per cent of mothers with a primary-level education and 19 per cent of those with medical cards attended antenatal classes before the birth of their last baby. It is interesting that partners attended classes with just one out of every four mothers. When asked about the doctor seen during antenatal visits, only 47 per cent of medical-card holders has seen the same doctor at each visit, compared with 69 per cent of those without medical cards. For one out of every two single mothers, parents were the main source of support after leaving the hospital and only 69 per cent of single mothers felt adequately prepared to go home with their baby. Following childbirth it is estimated that 38 per cent of all mothers had "baby blues", while 11 per cent had postnatal depression.

The majority of women have expressed a clear preference for longer maternity leave and the availability of paternity leave for fathers. An increase in the availability of crèche facilities in the work place is also the preference of the majority of women. Women in general believe that they need more preparation for parenting.

Recommendations

Given the importance of attendance at antenatal classes for the improvement of birth outcomes, it is essential that early attendance be encouraged and that all access and availability problems be removed to ensure that this service is available locally to all expectant mothers.

In keeping with the expressed preferences of Irish women, consideration should be given to ensuring that tests are routinely available in publicly funded hospitals, which can assess whether a baby has any abnormality prior to birth.

Every effort should be made to ensure that the preferences of the majority of women with medical cards to see the same doctor during the antenatal visits are satisfactorily fulfilled.

The "baby blues" and/or postnatal depression cause problems for a substantial proportion of women. Minimising the experience of these conditions and recognising them and treating them where they do occur should constitute a priority issue for antenatal services and postnatal care during the hospital stay and following discharge.

Given the preferences of the majority of women, greater flexibility in the length and funding of maternity leave and the introduction of paternity leave should be considered.

The necessity of increasing the availability of crèche facilities in the work place should be addressed as a matter of urgency.

More attention to the development of parenting skills should be considered for inclusion in antenatal and postnatal education programmes. Essential information like the safest sleeping position for the baby should be given to parents orally and in writing before discharge from hospital, or by the midwife in the case of home deliveries. Single women, in particular, have indicated a need for better preparation in learning to care for their babies. Additional support for this group might therefore need to be provided in antenatal classes, antenatal visits, during the hospital stay for delivery and during postnatal care following discharge.

Attitudes and Approaches to Breast-feeding

The findings in this study that the majority of mothers never breast-fed any of their babies supports the results forthcoming from previous research into the incidence of breast-feeding in Ireland. Mothers with higher levels of education, without medical cards and those who have attended antenatal classes are all more likely to choose breast-feeding rather than bottle feeding. When asked what would have helped them to continue breast-feeding, more than 10 per cent of mothers specified more help from the nurse or the health visitor. While the finding that three out of four mothers have never been made to feel embarrassed while breast-feeding is positive, this is moderated by the fact that facilities for breast-feeding in public places are considered by the majority of mothers to be inadequate.

Recommendations

Given the positive benefits for the health of the baby, the general objectives of the national policy on breast-feeding to increase the proportion of Irish mothers choosing to breast-feed should be actively supported. If this objective is to be achieved, the results of this study would suggest that education programmes and health promotion initiatives need to be targeted to expectant and new mothers (and their partners) in specific social circumstances. In particular, more effective channels of communication need to be used to convey the benefits of breast-feeding to women with fewer years of formal education, to those with medical cards and to those who do not attend antenatal classes. As the majority of these women tend to remain outside formal education structures after the minimum age, there may be good grounds for including in the school curriculum for young teenagers information programmes on the benefits of breast-feeding. The pursuit of this strategy would be consistent with previous research which has shown that the incidence of breast-feeding is positively influenced by early education on the benefits to the baby, and by the support of partners.

Conclusion

The information collected by the national survey of women's health needs constitutes the most valuable resource currently available on what Irish women do for their own health care, together with prevailing knowledge and attitudes regarding the health-care requirements of Irish women. While it is difficult to abstract some of the main findings from a data source as extensive as that analysed here, this study has attempted to do so with the objective of identifying those policy recommendations which may be most clearly indicated by these results. The pursuit of the policy recommendations presented here will require a range of responses from the policy-makers and service providers. In some areas — for example, improving the accessibility of family planning services and the incidence of breast-feeding — what is required is the active implementation of existing guidelines. For the achievement of other objectives — like the reduction of smoking among all women, and pregnant women in particular — more targeted and strategically managed health promotion policies will be required. It seems reasonable to conclude with regard to all the health promotion initiatives considered here that future policies should have specific regard to those women in most need and at greatest risk and who too frequently lack the essential information necessary for the achievement and maintenance of good health. In recognising that any new initiatives necessitated by the recommendations presented here will have to be considered in the context of the whole range of demands on health-care resources, the opportunities that might exist for re-directing currently available resources to areas yielding a better return on the investment might be worthy of serious consideration.

While the current commitment by government to the development of a national policy for women's health in Ireland is to be welcomed, the results of this study highlight the importance of on-going and widespread consultation with women in all sectors of society if this policy is to be well informed and truly responsive to the needs and aspirations of Irish women.

Appendix 1
Questionnaire

NATIONAL SURVEY OF WOMEN'S HEALTH NEEDS

April 1993

ID1

AREA CODE_____   ID CODE_____   ID2

INTERVIEWER NAME_____   INTVR. NO._____   INTVR

The National Maternity Hospital (Holles Street) is celebrating its centenary next year. To mark this event, it has asked the ESRI to carry out a national survey of women's health needs. Your name has been selected at random from the Electoral Register to participate in this survey. The women to be interviewed must all be aged between 18 and 60 years. **[INTVR: Check that the respondent fits into this age group.]** I would be very grateful if you would spend about 50 minutes talking to me about a range of issues related to women's health needs. All of the answers that you give will be treated in the strictest confidence by the ESRI, and only combined figures based on the answers of groups of women will be released to any person or body outside the ESRI. The results of the survey will be very important for planning future health services for women in Ireland.

SECTION 1 — NUTRITION

1. Do you think the food a woman eats *prior* to pregnancy affects her baby's health?

Yes	☐₁	
No	☐₂	
Don't know	☐₃	W1.1

2. Do you think the food a woman eats *during* pregnancy affects her baby's health?

Yes	☐₁	
No	☐₂	
Don't know	☐₃	W2.1

3. How often do you eat the following foods? (Tick one box on each line.)

	Every Day	3–4 Times a Week	Once a Week	Less Often	
Chips	☐₁	☐₂	☐₃	☐₄	W3.1
Fresh (not frozen) vegetables	☐₁	☐₂	☐₃	☐₄	W3.2
Fruit	☐₁	☐₂	☐₃	☐₄	W3.3

4. Are you a vegetarian?

Yes ☐₁ No ☐₂	W4.1

5. Which of the following foods are high in iron?

	High in iron	Not High in iron	Don't know	
Beef	☐₁	☐₂	☐₃	W5.1
Liver	☐₁	☐₂	☐₃	W5.2
Fish	☐₁	☐₂	☐₃	W5.3
Chicken	☐₁	☐₂	☐₃	W5.4

6. Which of the following foods are rich in calcium?

	Rich in calcium	Not rich in calcium	Don't know	
Cheese	☐₁	☐₂	☐₃	W6.1
Butter	☐₁	☐₂	☐₃	W6.2
Sardines	☐₁	☐₂	☐₃	W6.3
Yogurt	☐₁	☐₂	☐₃	W6.4

7. **Apart from milk in tea or coffee, how often do you take calcium-rich foods, i.e., milk or milk products?**

Every day	$\square_1$	
3–4 times weekly	$\square_2$	
Once weekly	$\square_3$	W7.1
Less often	$\square_4$	

8. **Regarding your weight, do you consider yourself:**

The right weight	$\square_1$	
Slightly overweight	$\square_2$	
Very overweight	$\square_3$	W8.1
Underweight	$\square_4$	

9. **Do you take any of the following products or preparations? If yes, how often? (Read out and tick all that apply)**

	Every Day	3–4 times weekly	Once weekly	Occasionally	Never	
Royal Jelly	$\square_1$	$\square_2$	$\square_3$	$\square_4$	$\square_5$	
Evening Primrose Oil	$\square_1$	$\square_2$	$\square_3$	$\square_4$	$\square_5$	W9.1
Cod Liver Oil	$\square_1$	$\square_2$	$\square_3$	$\square_4$	$\square_5$	W9.2
Vitamin supplements	$\square_1$	$\square_2$	$\square_3$	$\square_4$	$\square_5$	W9.3
Other	$\square_1$	$\square_2$	$\square_3$	$\square_4$	$\square_5$	W9.4

W9.5

Specify_____

___W9.6

10. **How often do you do physical activities of any kind lasting at least 20 minutes which make you short of breath and perspire, e.g., running, cycling, swimming, golf, gardening, etc?**

4 or more times per week	$\square_1$	
2–3 times per week	$\square_2$	
Once a week	$\square_3$	W10.1
Less than once a week	$\square_4$	
Never	$\square_5$	

11. **Do you believe that taking exercise in leisure time contributes towards better health?**

        Yes $\Box_1$

        No $\Box_2$ → Go to Q. 13   W11.1

        Don't know $\Box_3$ → Go to Q. 13

12. **Do you think you take enough exercise to stay healthy?**

        Yes $\Box_1$

        No $\Box_2$ W12.1

        Not sure $\Box_3$

        Please comment: _____ ___W12.2

13. **Would you like to take more exercise in your leisure time than you do at present?**

        Yes $\Box_1$

        No $\Box_2$ → Go to Q. 15   W13.1

        Not sure $\Box_3$ → Go to Q. 15

14. **Which, if any, of the reasons listed below prevents you from taking more exercise in leisure time? (Read out and tick one box on each line.)**

	Yes	No	
Work/Study commitments	$\Box_1$	$\Box_2$	W14.1
Tiredness after work/lectures	$\Box_1$	$\Box_2$	W14.2
Lack of money	$\Box_1$	$\Box_2$	W14.3
Lack of easily available facilities at work	$\Box_1$	$\Box_2$	W14.4
Lack of easily available facilities in the community	$\Box_1$	$\Box_2$	W14.5
Lack of interest of workmates/friends to go along	$\Box_1$	$\Box_2$	W14.6
Other	$\Box_1$	$\Box_2$	W14.7

Please specify:_____ ___W14.8

SECTION 2 — SEX EDUCATION

15. **Did you receive any sex education when you were growing up?**

        Yes   ☐₁

        No   ☐₂ → Go to Q. 18

W15.1

16. **If yes, where did you receive it? (Tick all that apply)**

    In School   ☐₁   W16.1

    From parents/guardian ☐₂   W16.2

    Friends/brother/sister ☐₃   W16.3

    Other   ☐₄   W16.4

    Specify_____ ___W16.5

17. **Overall, how adequate do you consider the sex education was that you received when you were growing up?**

    Completely adequate ☐₁

    Adequate   ☐₂

    Inadequate   ☐₃   W17.1

    Very inadequate   ☐₄

18. **Do you agree or disagree with the following statements:**

	Agree	Disagree	Don't know	
You cannot get pregnant while you are breast-feeding	☐₁	☐₂	☐₃	W18.1
You cannot get pregnant the first time you have sexual intercourse	☐₁	☐₂	☐₃	W18.2
You are most likely to get pregnant the first few days after your period	☐₁	☐₂	☐₃	W18.3
Women going through the change of life cannot get pregnant	☐₁	☐₂	☐₃	W18.4

19. **When is a woman most likely to become pregnant?**

        Beginning of her cycle   ❑₁

        Middle of her cycle   ❑₂   W19.1

        End of her cycle   ❑₃

        Don't know   ❑₄

SECTION 3 — SEXUALLY-TRANSMITTED DISEASES

20. **Who is particularly at risk of being infected with the AIDS virus? (DO NOT READ OUT, BUT PROBE FULLY ASKING "ANYONE ELSE?" AND CODE ALL THAT APPLY BELOW.)**

Those injecting drugs	❑₁	W20.1
Homosexuals/bisexuals	❑₂	W20.2
Those who have casual sex/several partners	❑₃	W20.3
Those who have sexual intercourse with a person		
infected with the AIDS virus	❑₄	W20.4
Unborn children of an infected woman	❑₅	W20.5
Haemophiliacs	❑₆	W20.6
Those receiving blood transfusions	❑₇	W20.7
Prostitutes	❑₈	W20.8
Other (specify)	❑₉	W20.9
_____		W20.10
Don't know	❑₁₀	__W20.11

21. **Given that sexual intercourse is a common method of spreading the AIDS virus, what do you think are the most effective things sexually-active people can do to reduce their risks? (DO NOT READ OUT, BUT PROMPT WITH "IS THERE ANYTHING ELSE THEY CAN DO?" AND TICK ALL THAT APPLY.)**

Stay with one partner	❑₁	W21.1
Reduce the number of partners they have	❑₂	W21.2
Use a condom	❑₃	W21.3
Abstain from sexual intercourse	❑₄	W21.4
Avoid casual sex	❑₅	W21.5
Use safe sex practices	❑₆	W21.6
Other (specify)	❑₇	W21.7
_____		
Don't know/no reply	❑₈	W21.8

SECTION 4 — FAMILY PLANNING

22. **Are you sexually active nowadays?**

    Yes   ☐₁

    No   ☐₂   → Go to Q. 26

    W22.1

23. **If yes, what method of family planning, if any, are you using at present? [INTVR: Code all mentioned. Do not read out list.]**

Natural	☐₁	Mini pill	☐₆
Coil/IUD	☐₂	Condom	☐₇
Diaphragm	☐₃	Spermicide	☐₈
Withdrawal	☐₄	Sterilisation	☐₉
Combined pill	☐₅	None	☐₁₀

    W23.1,6
    W23.2,7
    W23.3,8
    W23.4,9
    W23.5,10

24. **Have you used any other methods in the past?**

    Yes   ☐₁

    No   ☐₂   → Go to Q. 26

    W24.1

25. **If yes, why did you change?**
    [INTVR: Do not read out list. Tick all that apply.]

Failure, got pregnant	☐₁	Fear of pregnancy	☐₄
Made me feel sick	☐₂	Fear of side effects	☐₅
Difficulties in use	☐₃	Other	☐₆
		(Specify_____)	

    W25.1,4
    W25.2,5
    W25.3,6
    ___W25.7

26. **If you wanted it, where would you obtain information on family planning in your area? [INTVR: Code all mentioned. Do not read out list.]**

General practitioner	☐₁	Pharmacy	☐₆
Hospital	☐₂	Sister/Friends	☐₇
Health Centre	☐₃	Parents	☐₈
Family Planning Clinic	☐₄	Books/Magazines	☐₉
Public Health Nurse	☐₅	Other	☐₁₀
		(Specify_____)	

    W26.1,6
    W26.2,7
    W26.3,8
    W26.4,9
    W26.5,10
    W26.11

    Would not seek information locally on Family Planning   ☐₁₁

    W26.12

27. **Do you think the information you (would) receive on family planning in your area is (would be):**

        Completely adequate   ☐₁

        Adequate   ☐₂   W27.1

        Inadequate   ☐₃

        Very inadequate   ☐₄

28. **Do you think that family planning advice is easily accessible in your area?**

        Yes   ☐₁

        No   ☐₂   → Go to Q. 30   W28.1

        Don't know   ☐₃   → Go to Q. 30

29. **If yes, do you avail of this advice?**

        Yes ☐₁   No ☐₂   W29.1

30. **Where do you think family planning advice should be available? [INTVR: Code all mentioned. Do not read out list.]**

Hospital	☐₁	W30.1
Health Centre	☐₂	W30.2
GP	☐₃	W30.3
Public Health Nurse	☐₄	W30.4
Well Woman Clinic/Family Planning Clinic	☐₅	W30.5
Other	☐₆	W30.6
(Specify_____)		___W30.7

31. **(a) Do you think condoms should be sold in Ireland?**

        Yes, without a prescription   ☐₁

        Yes, only with a prescription   ☐₂   W31.1

        No, should not be sold at all   ☐₃ → Go to Q. 32

    (b) If yes, should they be sold in (Tick one box on each line.)

	Yes	No	
Chemists?	☐₁	☐₂	W31.2
Supermarkets?	☐₁	☐₂	W31.3
Any retail outlet that wants to stock them?	☐₁	☐₂	W31.4
Pubs, discos etc.?	☐₁	☐₂	W31.5

32. **Do you think that sterilisation should be available to (a) women and (b) men in all publicly funded hospitals?**

	Yes	*No*	*Don't know*	
(a) Women	❏₁	❏₂	❏₃	W32.1
(b) Men	❏₁	❏₂	❏₃	W32.2

SECTION 5 — MATERNITY LEAVE

33. **Have you had a baby, while in paid employment, since 1975?**

Yes ❏₁   No ❏₂ → Go to Q. 36   W33.1

34. **If yes, did you avail of maternity leave?**

Yes ❏₁

No, did not qualify ❏₂ → Go to Q. 36   W34.1

No, gave up work ❏₃ → Go to Q. 36

35. **If yes, do you think that your maternity leave was adequate?**

Yes ❏₁   No ❏₂   W35.1

ASK ALL

36. **If you were pregnant and had a choice, which of the following would you prefer?**

14 weeks' maternity leave with full pay ❏₁

6 months with half pay ❏₂

One year without pay ❏₃   W36.1

37. **Do you think that fathers should receive paid paternity leave?**

Yes ❏₁   No ❏₂ → Go to Q. 39   W37.1

38. **If yes, how much paternity leave do you feel would be appropriate?**

One week ❏₁

Two weeks ❏₂

More than 3 weeks ❏₃

Other ❏₄ (Specify_____)   W38.1

39. INTVR: Ask if in paid employment: Are crèche facilities available at your place of employment?

        Yes $\square_1$ No $\square_2$→ Go to Q. 41

W39.1

40. If yes, do/did you use this facility?

        Yes $\square_1$ No $\square_2$ No, pre-school children $\square_3$

W40.1

41. ASK ALL: Do you think crèche facilities should be provided in the work place?

        Yes $\square_1$ No $\square_2$→ Go to Q. 43

W41.1

42. If yes, how do you think they should be funded?

By the state	$\square_1$ By state and parents	$\square_5$
By the employer	$\square_2$ By employer and parents	$\square_6$
By parents	$\square_3$ By combination of all three	$\square_7$
By state and employer $\square_4$	Don't know	$\square_8$

W42.1

SECTION 6 — HOSPITAL SERVICES FOR MOTHERS

Sub-section 1 — Antenatal Education

43. (a) Have you ever had a baby?

        Yes $\square_1$ No $\square_2$→ Go to Q. 80

W43.1

(b) IF YES: How many babies have you had?

        Number_____

W43.2

(c) What age were you when you had a) your first baby and b) your last baby?

        First baby_____   Last baby_____

W43.3

(d) Did you ever (intentionally) give birth to a baby at home?

        Yes $\square_1$ → Go to Q. 44   No $\square_2$

W43.4

(e) IF NO: Would you have liked to give birth at home?

        Yes $\square_1$ No $\square_2$

W43.5

NOW I WOULD LIKE TO ASK YOU SOME QUESTIONS ABOUT YOUR EXPERIENCE WITH THE BIRTH OF YOUR *LAST* BABY.

44. **(a) With regard to antenatal care, which of the following did you mainly attend?**

   Public hospital clinic $\square_1$

   Semi-private clinic $\square_2$ W44.1

   Private clinic/rooms $\square_3$

   Other $\square_4$ ___W44.2

   (Specify_____)

 (b) In relation to these antenatal visits, would you say you had enough time with your doctor or midwife at each visit?

   Yes $\square_1$ No $\square_2$ W44.3

45. **Did you feel you had enough privacy at your visits?**

               W45.1

   Yes $\square_1$ No $\square_2$

46. **(If respondent was in paid employment when pregnant) Did taking time off for your antenatal visits/classes present a problem for you in your work place?**

               W46.1

   Yes $\square_1$ No $\square_2$ Was not at work $\square_3$

47. **(a) Did you always see the same doctor/midwife at each visit?**

   Yes $\square_1$ No $\square_2$ W47.1

 (b) If no, would you have liked to have seen the same doctor/midwife at each visit?

               W47.2

   Yes $\square_1$ No $\square_2$ Don't mind $\square_3$

48. **(a) At what time of day did you usually attend for antenatal care? [Code one answer in first column below.]**

 (b) What time of day would have been most convenient to you? [Code one answer in second column below.]

	Usually	*Most Convenient*	
Morning	$\square_1$	$\square_1$	
Lunch time	$\square_2$	$\square_2$	W48.1
Afternoon	$\square_3$	$\square_3$	W48.2
Evening	$\square_4$	$\square_4$	

49. **During the course of your antenatal visits, did you feel the following personnel showed sufficient interest in your concerns?**

	Yes	No	Not Applicable	
Doctors	☐₁	☐₂	—	W49.1
Nurses	☐₁	☐₂	—	W49.2
Social Workers	☐₁	☐₂	☐₃	W49.3
Physiotherapists	☐₁	☐₂	☐₃	W49.4

50. **Did you attend antenatal classes in preparation for childbirth?**

   Yes ☐₁ → Go to Q. 52   No ☐₂   W50.1

51. **If not, why not? [INTVR: Do not read out list, but prompt with "Is there anything else?", and tick all that apply.]**

Too far away	☐₁	W51.1
Too costly	☐₂	W51.2
No time	☐₃	W51.3
No baby minders	☐₄ Go to Q. 55	W51.4
Did them before	☐₅	W51.5
Don't think they are of any use	☐₆	W51.6
Other	☐₇	W51.7
(Specify_____)		W51.8
Don't know	☐₈	___W51.9

52. **Where did you attend?**

Hospital	☐₁	
Health Centre	☐₂	W52.1
Privately	☐₃	
Other	☐₄	
(Specify_____)		___W52.2

53. **Did the classes prepare you adequately for the birth?**

Very well	☐₁	
Adequately	☐₂	W53.1
Inadequately	☐₃	
Very Inadequately	☐₄	

54. Did your partner attend classes with you?

       Yes   ❑₁

       No   ❑₂   W54.1

       No partner   ❑₃

55. Should tests be available in Irish hospitals to show if a baby has any abnormality before it is born?

       Yes   ❑₁

       No   ❑₂   W55.1

       Don't know   ❑₃

Sub-section 2 — Postnatal

56. Thinking of your last baby, how long were you in hospital after delivery?

              _____days   W56.1

57. Was this postnatal stay long enough?

       Yes ❑₁ → Go to Q. 59   No ❑₂   W57.1

58. If no, what would you consider an adequate stay?
              _____days   W58.1

59. Did you feel you were adequately prepared for going home with your baby?

       Yes ❑₁ → Go to Q. 61   No ❑₂   W59.1

60. If no, from whom would you like to have received further support?
[INTVR: Do not read out list.]

       GP   ❑₁   W60.1

       Public Health Nurse ❑₂   W60.2

       Obstetrician   ❑₃   W60.3

       Midwife   ❑₄   W60.4

       Mother/relative/friend ❑₅   W60.5

       Other   ❑₆   W60.6

       (Specify_____)   ___W60.7

61. **Who gave you the most help and support when you got home with your baby? [INTVR: Do not read out list.]**

Partner	☐₁	Hospital Staff	☐₆	W61.1,6
Sister/brother (in-law)	☐₂	Nurse/Public Health Visitor	☐₇	W61.2,7
Parent (in-law)	☐₃	La Leche/Irish Childbirth Trust	☐₈	W61.3,8
Friend/neighbour	☐₄	Other	☐₉	W61.4,9
GP	☐₅	(Specify_____)		W61.5
				W61.10

62. **What effect, if any, did the arrival of the new baby have on your relationship with your partner? [INTVR: Do not read out list.]**

Relationship improved   ☐₁

Relationship disimproved   ☐₂   W62.1

No great change   ☐₃

Not relevant — no partner   ☐₄

63. **Do you think your partner felt neglected or left out?**

Yes   ☐₁

No   ☐₂   W63.1

Don't know   ☐₃

Not relevant — no partner   ☐₄

64. **Following the birth of any of your babies, have you ever suffered from the following:**

Postnatal depression to the extent that you

    needed medical help   ☐₁

Baby blues (felt down for a few days)   ☐₂   W64.1

Never felt at all depressed   ☐₃

SECTION 7 — BREAST-FEEDING

65. **Did you breast-feed:**

First baby   ☐₁

Some of your babies   ☐₂

All of your babies   ☐₃   W65.1

Never breast-fed   ☐₄ → Go to Q. 72

66. **Why did you decide to breast-feed?**
    [Tick all mentioned.]

Best for baby	☐₁	W66.1
Convenience	☐₂	W66.2
Economical	☐₃	W66.3
Recover figure	☐₄	W66.4
		W66.5
Other	☐₅ (Specify_____)	W66.6

67. **Thinking of your last breast-fed baby, for how long did you breast-feed?**

Less than 6 weeks	☐₁	
3 months	☐₂	
More than 3 months but less than 6 months	☐₃	W67.1
Longer	☐₄	

68. **Why did you stop breast-feeding?**
    [Do not read out, but prompt with "Any other reason?" and tick all mentioned.]

Went back to work	☐₁	Baby got teeth	☐₇	W68.1,7
Difficult to do it in social situations	☐₂	Baby old enough to drink from cup	☐₈	W68.2,8
Didn't like it	☐₃	Felt it was time to stop	☐₉	W68.3,9
Too demanding	☐₄	Breast problems	☐₁₀	W68.4,10
Baby not settling	☐₅	Other	☐₁₁	W68.5,11
Baby not getting enough	☐₆	(Specify_____)		W68.6 __W68.12

69. **If you stopped because of difficulties, who/what would have helped you to continue?**

_____ __W69.1

_____ __W69.2

_____ __W69.3

70. **Have you ever been made feel embarrassed while breast-feeding?**

Yes ☐₁ No ☐₂		W70.1

71. **Did you think that facilities in public places are adequate for breast-feeding mothers?**

    Yes ☐₁   No ☐₂   Don't know ☐₃   W71.1

72. **Is it all right for a woman to take the pill while breast-feeding?**

    Yes ☐₁   No ☐₂   Don't know ☐₃   W72.1

SECTION 8 — PARENTING SKILLS

73. **Would you have liked more preparation for parenting?**

    Yes ☐₁   No ☐₂   Don't know ☐₃   W73.1

74. **What problems, if any, have you had with your last baby? [Do not read out, but prompt with "Anything else?", and tick all mentioned.]**

Sore eyes	☐₁	Nappy rash ☐₇	W74.1,7
Cradle cap	☐₂	Snuffles ☐₈	W74.2,8
Feeding	☐₃	Vomiting ☐₉	W74.3,9
Crying	☐₄	Diarrhoea ☐₁₀	W74.4,10
Sleeplessness	☐₅	Other ☐₁₁ (Specify_____)	W74.5,11
Not sure how to feed ☐₆		No problems ☐₁₂ → Go to Q. 77	W74.6,12
			W74.13

75. **If you had any problems with your baby, from whom, if anyone, did you receive help? [Do not read out, but prompt with "Anyone else?", and tick all mentioned.]**

GP	☐₁	Family ☐₇	W75.1,7
Public Health Nurse	☐₂	Friends ☐₈	W75.2,8
Nurse in GP Surgery	☐₃	Other ☐₉	W75.3,9
Health Centre	☐₄	Was able to manage on my own ☐₁₀	W75.4,10
Hospital Doctor/Nurse	☐₅	Did not get any help ☐₁₁	W75.5,11
Partner	☐₆	Did not know where to go for help ☐₁₂	W75.6,12

76. **If you sought help from a doctor or nurse were you satisfied with the help you received?**

	Yes	*No*	
Doctor	$\square_1$	$\square_2$	W76.1
Nurse	$\square_1$	$\square_2$	W76.2

77. **If you have more than one child, have you experienced a lot of jealousy and competition between the other children and the new baby?**

Yes $\square_1$

No $\square_2$ → Go to Q. 79

Have only one child $\square_3$ → Go to Q. 79

Don't know $\square_4$ → Go to Q. 79   W77.1

78. **If yes, what can be done to help with this?**
[Do not read out, but prompt with "Anything else?", and tick all mentioned.]

Get new baby to buy present for children	$\square_1$	W78.1
Give other children extra attention and love	$\square_2$	W78.2
Involve other children in helping with new baby	$\square_3$	W78.3
Slap or give telling off	$\square_4$	W78.4
Other (Specify_____)	$\square_5$	W78.5
Don't know	$\square_6$	W78.6
		___W78.7

79. **Which of these positions is safest for a sleeping baby?**
[Tick one box only]

On back $\square_1$

On side $\square_2$ W79.1

On stomach $\square_3$

SECTION 9 — GYNAECOLOGY

80. **Have you ever attended a gynaecologist or gynaecological clinic for any reason apart from antenatal care during a pregnancy?**

Yes $\square_1$ No $\square_2$→ Go to Q. 82   W80.1

81. **If yes, why? [Do not read out but tick all mentioned.]**

Heavy periods	☐₁	Urinary Problems	☐₇		W81.1,6
Irregular bleeding	☐₂	Endometriosis	☐₈		W81.2,7
Prolapse	☐₃	Ovarian Cysts	☐₉		W81.3,8
Family Planning	☐₄	Infertility	☐₁₀		W81.4,9
Smear	☐₅	Sexual Problems	☐₁₁		W81.5,10
Amenorrhea	☐₆	Other	☐₁₂		W81.11
		(Specify_____)			_W81.12

82. **How frequently should a woman have a smear?**

Once a year ☐₁
Every two years ☐₂
Every three years ☐₃   W82.1
Less often ☐₄
Don't know ☐₅

83. **Have you yourself ever had a cervical smear?**

Yes ☐₁   No ☐₂→ Go to Q. 86   W83.1

84. **How long is it since you had your last smear?**

Less than 12 months ☐₁
1–2 years ☐₂   W84.1
2–3 years ☐₃
More than 3 years ☐₄

85. **Have you ever had an abnormal cervical smear?**

Yes ☐₁   No ☐₂   W85.1

86. **Has anyone in your family had an abnormal smear?**

Yes ☐₁   No ☐₂   W86.1

87. **Has any close female relative in your family had cancer of the cervix?**

Yes ☐₁   No ☐₂   W87.1

88. **Which of the following (male or female) would you pre-fer to attend for a smear? (Tick one box only)**

	Male	Female
Gynaecologist	$\Box_1$	$\Box_8$
GP	$\Box_2$	$\Box_9$
Family Planning Clinic Nurse	$\Box_3$	$\Box_{10}$
Family Planning Doctor	$\Box_4$	$\Box_{11}$
Hospital Nurse	$\Box_5$	$\Box_{12}$
Community Nurse	$\Box_6$	$\Box_{13}$
Nurse in GP surgery	$\Box_7$	$\Box_{14}$

W88.1

89. **Do you perform routine self-examination of your breasts?**

Frequently $\Box_1$ → Go to Q. 91

Occasionally $\Box_2$ → Go to Q. 91 W89.1

Never $\Box_3$

90. **If not, why?**
[INTVR: Do not read out list, but tick all mentioned.]

Afraid of what I would find $\Box_1$ W90.1

Find it embarrassing $\Box_2$ W90.2

Don't know what to do $\Box_3$ W90.3

Doctor does it $\Box_4$ W90.4

Don't think it is any use $\Box_5$ W90.5

No particular reason $\Box_6$ W90.6

Other $\Box_7$ (Specify_____) W90.7 W90.8

Don't know $\Box_8$ ___W90.9

91. **What time in the month, in relation to your period, is the best time to carry out a breast examination?**

The week following the period $\Box_1$ W91.1

Other $\Box_2$ (Specify_____) ___W91.2

Don't know $\Box_3$

92. **Which women should have a mammogram (breast x-ray)? [INTVR: Do not read out list.]**

Those under 30 years	❑₁	W92.1
Those over 30 years	❑₂	W92.2
		W92.3
Those over 40 years	❑₃	W92.4
Those over 50 years	❑₄	
Those who have had a close female relative with breast cancer	❑₅	W92.5
Those who have had breast lumps or other worrying changes in the breast	❑₆	W92.6
		W92.7
Other	❑₇ (Specify_____)	___W92.8

93. **Has any close female relative of yours had breast cancer? (e.g. mother, maternal grandmother, sister, daughter)**

Yes ❑₁   No ❑₂   Don't know ❑₃   W93.1

94. **Have you a preference in relation to who carries out a breast examination for you?**

Male doctor	❑₁	W94.1
Female doctor	❑₂	
Don't mind whether doctor is male or female	❑₃	
Other	❑4 (Specify_____)	___W94.2

95. **What are the symptoms of the onset of the menopause? [Tick all mentioned.]**

Hot flushes	❑₁	W95.1
Night sweats	❑₂	W95.2
		W95.3
Irritability	❑₃	W95.4
Irregular periods/periods stop	❑₄	W95.5
Other	❑₅ (Specify_____)	W95.6
Don't know	❑₆	___W95.7

96. **Do you feel you have/or can get adequate information on the menopause?**

Yes ❑₁   No ❑₂   Don't know ❑₃ | W96.1

97. **From whom would you seek information on the meno-pause? [Tick all mentioned.]**

GP	❑₁	W97.1
Gynaecologist	❑₂	W97.2
Nurse	❑₃	W97.3
Health Centre	❑₄	W97.4
Books/Magazines/Video	❑₅	W97.5
Friends/Family	❑₆	W97.6
Health Promotion Unit	❑₇	W97.7
Family Planning Clinic	❑₈	W97.8
Other	❑₉ (Specify_____)	W97.9
		__W97.10

98. **Why do women sometimes have hormone replacement therapy prescribed?**
    [INTVR: Do not read out list. Tick all mentioned.]

To relieve the symptoms of the menopause	❑₁	W98.1
To relieve the symptoms of osteoporosis	❑₂	W98.2
Following a total hysterectomy	❑₃	W98.3
Other	❑₄ (Specify_____)	W98.4
Don't know	❑₅	W98.5
		__W98.6

99. **Have you ever, taken or are you now taking, hormone replacement therapy (HRT)?**

Yes ❑₁ → Go to Q. 86   No ❑₂ | W99.1

100. **If no, would you consider taking hormone replacement therapy during the menopause?**

Yes ❑₁   No ❑₂   Don't know ❑₃ | W100.1

101. What is osteoporosis?

Thinning of the bones ☐₁   Other/Don't know ☐₃ | W101.1

102. Osteoporosis is a gradual thinning of the bones. Have you ever heard that any particular group of people is most at risk from this? Which group?
[INTVR: do not prompt. Tick one box only.]

Young women   ☐₁

Middle-aged and older women   ☐₂

Children   ☐₃
                                              W102.1
Men   ☐₄

Old people   ☐₅

Other   ☐₆ (Specify_____) _W102.2

Don't know   ☐₇

103. What are the causes of osteoporosis?
[INTVR: do not prompt. Tick all mentioned.]

Lack of oestrogen due to menopause ☐₁	W103.1
	W103.2
Lack of calcium in the bones ☐₂	W103.3
Arthritis ☐₃	W103.4
Lack of exercise ☐₄	W103.5
Overweight ☐₅	W103.6
Other ☐₆ (Specify_____)	W103.7
Don't know ☐₇	_W103.8

104. How can osteoporosis be avoided?
[INTVR: do not read out, but tick all mentioned.]

By taking hormone replacement therapy ☐₁	W104.1
By taking exercise ☐₂	W104.2
By taking a diet high in calcium (e.g. cheese and milk products)☐₃	W104.3
	W104.4
Other ☐₄ (Specify_____)	W104.5
Don't know ☐₅	_W104.6

105. Have you ever experienced unavoidable leaking of urine?

Yes ☐₁   No ☐₂→ Go to Q. 110   W105.1

106. If yes, is it nowadays a problem for you?

Yes ☐₁   No ☐₂→ Go to Q. 110   W106.1

107. Have you ever sought help or advice about this problem?

Yes ☐₁   No ☐₂→ Go to Q. 109   W107.1

108. If yes, from whom? [INTVR: do not prompt.]

GP	☐₁	Friends/Family	☐₅	W108.1,5
Nurse in GP Surgery	☐₂	Books/Magazines	☐₆	W108.2,6
Public Health Nurse	☐₃	Other	☐₇	W108.3,7
Hospital Staff	☐₄	(Specify_____)		W108.4
				_W108.8

109. If no, why not? [INTVR: do not prompt.]

Too embarrassed	☐₁	W109.1
Did not know where to get help	☐₂	W109.2
Did not know anything could be done	☐₃	W109.3
Learned to live with it	☐₄	W109.4
Other	☐₅ (Specify_____)	W109.5
		W109.6

110. Have you ever suffered from pre-menstrual tension, e.g., not feeling well before your period?

Yes ☐₁   No ☐₂→ Go to Q. 112   W110.1

111. If yes, what did you do to relieve the symptoms? [INTVR: Do not read out but tick all mentioned.]

Pain killers	☐₁	Alcohol	☐₆	W111.1,6
Hot baths	☐₂	Stayed in bed	☐₇	W111.2,7
Herbal remedies	☐₃	Suffered symptoms	☐₈	W111.3,8
Exercise	☐₄	Other	☐₉	W111.4,9
Hot water bottle	☐₅	(Specify_____)		W111.5
				_W111.10

SECTION 10 — FAMILY SIZE

112. What do you think is the ideal number of children to have in a family?_____   W112.1

113. How many children do you realistically think you are likely to have in your completed family?

None	$\Box_1$	4	$\Box_5$
1	$\Box_2$	5	$\Box_6$
2	$\Box_3$	6 or more	$\Box_7$
3	$\Box_4$		

W113.1

114. For those who give different answers to the two previous questions, ask: Why is there a difference between your ideal family size and the number of children you have or think you are likely to have in your completed family? [INTVR: Do not prompt.]

Partner wanted more children than I did $\Box_1$

Partner wanted fewer children than I did $\Box_2$

Contraception failure $\Box_3$

Can't have any children $\Box_4$

Can't have any more children $\Box_5$

Can't afford any more children $\Box_6$

Other $\Box_7$

Don't know $\Box_8$

W114.1

SECTION 11 — LIFESTYLES

115. Which of the following statements is true for you?

I smoke cigarettes regularly
(at least 1 per day every day) $\Box_1$

I smoke cigarettes occasionally $\Box_2 \rightarrow$ Go to Q. 117

I am an ex-smoker $\Box_3 \rightarrow$ Go to Q. 118

I have never smoked $\Box_4 \rightarrow$ Go to Q. 120

W115.1

116. How many cigarettes do you usually smoke per day?

1–5	$\square_1$	
6–10	$\square_2$	W116.1
11–19	$\square_3$	
20 or more	$\square_4$	

117. Would you like to give up smoking?

Yes $\square_1$ No $\square_2$ Don't know $\square_3$ W117.1

118. If you have ever been pregnant, did you smoke during any of your pregnancies?

Yes	$\square_1$	
No	$\square_2$	
Can't remember	$\square_3$	W118.1
Never been pregnant	$\square_4$	

119. If you were to become pregnant in the future, would you smoke during your pregnancy?

Yes $\square_1$ No $\square_2$ Don't know $\square_3$ W119.1

120. Could you tell me whether you agree or disagree with the following statements?

	Agree	Disagree	Don't know	
Smoking increases the risk of lung cancer	$\square_1$	$\square_2$	$\square_3$	W120.1
Smoking increases the risk of heart disease	$\square_1$	$\square_2$	$\square_3$	W120.2
Smoking increases the risk of bronchitis	$\square_1$	$\square_2$	$\square_3$	W120.3
If a pregnant woman smokes, her unborn baby smokes too	$\square_1$	$\square_2$	$\square_3$	W120.4
Smoking increases the risk of narrowing of the arteries in the legs which may lead to severe pain and gangrene	$\square_1$	$\square_2$	$\square_3$	W120.5

121. Can you tell me which of the following describes you?

A person who takes a drink $\square_1$

An ex-drinker $\square_2$→ Go to Q. 126

A person who has never taken alcohol $\square_3$→ Go to Q. 128   W121.1

122. If you drink alcohol, what would you most commonly drink? (Tick one box only.)

Beer $\square_1$

Cider $\square_2$

Wine $\square_3$

Spirits $\square_4$

Other $\square_5$ W122.1

123. How much of this drink do you generally have at any one time?

	None	*1*	*2*	*3*	*4*	*5*	*6/more*	
Glasses/Bottles or Shots (spirits)	$\square_1$	$\square_2$	$\square_3$	$\square_4$	$\square_5$	$\square_6$	$\square_7$	W123.1

124. On average, how many times in the past 12 months have you had enough drink to make you feel intoxicated?

None in the past 12 months	$\square_1$	2–3 times a month	$\square_6$
Once or twice	$\square_2$	1–2 times a week	$\square_7$
3–5 times in past 12 months	$\square_3$	3–4 times a week	$\square_8$
6–10 times in past 12 months	$\square_4$	5–6 times a week	$\square_9$
About once a month	$\square_5$	Every day	$\square_{10}$

W124.1

125. Why do you usually drink?
[INTVR: do not read out, but prompt with "Any other reason?" and tick all mentioned.]

To be sociable	$\square_1$	To cope with family stress	$\square_5$	W125.1,5
I enjoy a drink	$\square_2$	To cope with work stress	$\square_6$	W125.2,6
To relax	$\square_3$	Other	$\square_7$	W125.3,7
To cope with depression	$\square_4$	Don't know	$\square_8$	W125.4,8

126. If you have ever been pregnant, did you drink alcohol during the pregnancy?

I continued drinking as usual	$\square_1$	
I cut down	$\square_2$	
I gave up drinking	$\square_3$	
Have never been pregnant	$\square_4$	W126.1

127. If you were to become pregnant in the future, would you:

Continue drinking as usual $\square_1$

Cut down $\square_2$

Give up drinking $\square_3$ W127.1

Not relevant (not likely to become pregnant, too old, etc.) $\square_4$

128. Have you ever been on tranquillisers to help you cope with stress?

Yes $\square_1$ No $\square_2 \rightarrow$ Go to Q. 131   W128.1

129. If yes, how long were you on them?

Less than 1 month	$\square_1$	
1–2 months	$\square_2$	
2–3 months	$\square_3$	W129.1
More than 3 months	$\square_4$	

130. What was the particular cause of the stress at the time? [INTVR: Do not prompt. Tick one box only.]

Marital problems/ broken love affair	$\square_1$	Bereavement in family	$\square_5$	
Problems with children	$\square_2$	Inability to cope with personal illness	$\square_6$	
Financial problems	$\square_3$	Loneliness	$\square_7$	
Work problems	$\square_4$	Other (Specify_____)	$\square_8$	W130.1 _W130.2

**131. (a) What do you consider to have been the most stress-
ful event in your life? [INTVR: Do not prompt. Tick
one box only.]**

Loss of job (self)	☐₁	Rearing children	☐₁₀
Loss of job (husband)	☐₂	Husband's drinking problem	☐₁₁
Promotion	☐₃	Gambling	☐₁₂
Examinations	☐₄	A birth	☐₁₃
Moving house	☐₅	A death	☐₁₄
Financial matters	☐₆	Illness of my own	☐₁₅
Love affair	☐₇	Illness of family member	☐₁₆
Getting married	☐₈	Family conflict	☐₁₇
Marital problems	☐₉	No stressful event ☐₁₈ → Go to Q. 133	
		Other	☐₁₉
		(Specify_____)	

W131.1

_W131.2

**(b) How did you cope with this stressful event?
[INTVR: Do not prompt]**

_____

_____

_W131.3
_W131.4

**132. [SHOW CARD A] Apart from the ways you have men-
tioned above, here are some ways other people have
said they coped with a stressful event. Would any of
these apply to you?**

Talked to friends	☐₁	Prayed	☐₉	W132.1,9
Talked to family/partner	☐₂	Talked to doctor/nurse	☐₁₀	W132.2,10
Support group	☐₃	Cried	☐₁₁	W132.3,11
Went on spending spree	☐₄	Took up yoga	☐₁₂	W132.4,12
Went on a holiday	☐₅	Took tranquillisers/ sleeping pills	☐₁₃	W132.5,13
Went off alone to think	☐₆	Went for psychological counselling	☐₁₄	W132.6,14
Ate more	☐₇	Talked to priest/minister	☐₁₅	W132.7,15
Drank more alcohol	☐₈	Other	☐₁₆	W132.8,16
		(Specify_____)		_W132.17

133. (a) **Sometimes women are injured in various ways such as being beaten, raped, attacked with a weapon or threatened with death either by strangers or by people they know? Has anything like this ever happened to you? Please think carefully and remember that everything you say to me will be treated in the strictest confidence. If something like this has happened to you, how often would you say it happened?**

Never	$\square_1 \rightarrow$ Go to Q. 134	
Once	$\square_2$	
A few times	$\square_3$	W133.1
5–10 times	$\square_4$	
More than 10 times	$\square_5$	

(b) **Thinking of the last occasion this happened, was it**

In your own home? $\square_1$ Not in your own home? $\square_2$ | W133.2

(c) **Was it carried out by**

Someone you knew? $\square_1$ Someone you didn't know? $\square_2$ | W133.3

134. **Marital status of respondent**

Married	$\square_1$	Married but living apart (not legally separated or divorced) $\square_6$
Cohabiting with male in a stable relationship	$\square_2$	Divorced/ Legally Separated $\square_7$
Cohabiting with female in a stable relationship	$\square_3$	Widowed $\square_8$
Single but in a steady relationship	$\square_4$	W134.1
Single and not in a steady relationship	$\square_5$	

135. In relation to employment, could you describe your situation at present?

At work full time(30 hours + weekly) ☐₁   Student   ☐₆

At work part time (less than 30   Retired   ☐₇
   hours weekly)   ☐₂

At work as relative assisting   ☐₃   Ill/disabled   ☐₈

Unemployed   ☐₄   Others not in
                                   labour force   ☐₉

Engaged in home duties   ☐₅   W135.1

If not working [codes 4–9]: Are you looking for work?

      Yes ☐₁   No ☐₂   W135.2

136. What is your year of birth?   19___
                                                            W136.1

137. (a)   Are you covered by a Medical Card?   Yes ☐₁ No ☐₂
     (b)   Are you a member of VHI?   Yes ☐₁ No ☐₂ W137.1

W137.2

138. (a) (If ever engaged in paid work.) What is (was) your (last) occupation? [Please describe fully. If farmer, state acreage.]

_____

_____
                                                            _W138.1

(b) (If ever married or cohabiting.) What is (was) your partner's occupation? [Please describe fully. If farmer, state acreage.]

_____

_____
                                                            _W138.2

139. What is the highest level of education that you reached?

Got Primary Cert/no   Got qualification
   second-level examination ☐₁   from RTC etc.   ☐₄

Got Inter/Group/Junior   Got qualification
   Cert   ☐₂   from university   ☐₅

Got Leaving Cert/Matric   ☐₃
                                                            W139.1

Appendix 2
Women's Health Needs
Information Sheet

Thank you very much for participating in this survey. It is one of the most extensive pieces of research ever undertaken into the health needs of Irish women. As part of the study, some 3,000 women throughout the country are being interviewed. The results of the survey will have an important influence on the planning of future health services for women in Ireland.

The ESRI was commissioned to carry out the survey by The National Maternity Hospital at Holles Street. They are celebrating their centenary next year, and the results of the survey will be published as part of their celebrations. The ESRI was founded in 1960 in order to carry out research of relevance to Irish economic and social development. Your name was selected at random from the Register of Electors. All of the information that you gave in the interview will be treated in the strictest confidence by the ESRI, and only results based on the responses of groups of women will be published. Information on individual respondents will *never under any circumstances* be released to any external body.

If you would like more information on the survey in which you have participated, please contact **Miriam Murphy at the ESRI, phone (01) 676 0155**.[1]

Help and support for women who experience violence or abuse in their own home is provided by **Women's Aid**. This organisation can be contacted at **(01) 754121**.[2]

As you are aware, the survey covered a wide range of issues relevant to the health of women. Whereas some questions asked about your attitudes or opinions on a particular topic, a certain amount of information would have been required to answer some of the other questions. Some notes on these topics, which you might find useful, are given over the page.

---

[1] At the time of publication, the ESRI number is (01) 667 1525.

[2] At the time of publication, the Women's Aid number is 1800 34 19 00.

NUTRITION

A number of questions in the survey listed different foods, and you were asked about their iron and calcium content. Iron is very important for healthy blood. Foods that are high in iron include beef and liver. Fish and chicken are not high in iron. Calcium is essential for the development and maintenance of strong bones and teeth. Cheese, sardines and yogurt are all foods that are rich in calcium. Butter is not rich in calcium.

SEX EDUCATION

In the section on sex education, some statements were read out to you describing situations where a woman might or might not become pregnant. A woman *can* become pregnant while she is breast-feeding and the first time she has sexual intercourse. Also, women going through the change of life *can* get pregnant. A woman is most likely to become pregnant in the middle of her cycle.

BREAST-FEEDING

It is quite safe for a woman to take the contraceptive pill while breast-feeding *provided* that it is the mini-pill. The combined oral contraceptive pill should not be taken while breast-feeding.

PARENTING

The safest position for a sleeping baby is on his/her side.

GYNAECOLOGICAL ISSUES

A large part of the survey dealt with gynaecological matters. There were several questions on **Cervical Smear** tests — also known as **PAP Smears**. A smear test involves gently scraping the cervix with a small wooden spatula to obtain a sample of cells, which are then examined in a laboratory. It is recommended that all women have a smear test every 2/3 years.

Routine self-examination of breasts should also be carried out by all women. The week following a period is the best time of the month to carry out a breast examination. As well, women who have had breast lumps or other worrying changes in the breast, and women who have had a close female relative with breast cancer, should have a mammogram — i.e., a breast x-ray. It is also advisable for any women aged over 50 years to have a mammogram.

The issue of **Hormone Replacement Therapy (HRT)** was also covered in the survey. This involves replacement of the hormone oestrogen. This hormone is normally present in a woman's body up to the time her ovaries stop functioning. HRT is prescribed to relieve the symptoms of the menopause and osteoporosis. It is also prescribed following a total hysterectomy.

Some questions were also asked about **Osteoporosis**. This condition can be described as a gradual thinning of the bones. Middle-aged and older women, and old people in general, are particularly at risk from osteoporosis. It is caused by a lack of calcium in the bones, lack of oestrogen due to the menopause and also by lack of exercise. It can best be avoided by taking a diet that is high in calcium-rich foods (e.g. cheese and milk products), taking Hormone Replacement Therapy, and by exercising regularly.

Appendix 3
Results of Logistic Regression Analysis

Table A1: Analysis of Smoking Intention During a Future Pregnancy for Women of Child-bearing Age who Smoke[†]

Effect		Estimate*	Standard Error	Chi-Square	Prob
		Logistic Regression Results			
Intercept		-0.9883	0.1331	55.17	0.0000
Medical-Card Status	Yes	0.2434	0.0826	8.67	0.0032
Employment Status	Full-time	-0.4569	0.1757	6.76	0.0093
	Part-time	-0.5155	0.2704	3.63	0.0566
	Unemployed	0.5228	0.2498	4.38	0.0364
	Home Duties	0.2363	0.1484	2.54	0.1113
Urban/Rural	Rural	-0.2697	0.0807	11.18	0.0008

† The levels of the dependent variable in this model are "Would/would not smoke during a future pregnancy". "Would smoke" is the first category and therefore the category for which the model predicts probabilities; those for the second category "Would not smoke" are calculated by subtraction.

* The sum of the parameter estimates for a combination of characteristics yields the logit of the probability from which the probabilities associated with each level of the response variable can be calculated. Under the modelling process used, the parameter estimates sum to zero for each independent variable. Therefore the estimates for the levels of the independent variables not reported to the table (not having a medical card, the "Other" employment category and living in an urban area) are calculated by subtraction.

Table A2: Analysis of Smoking Intention During a Future Pregnancy for Mothers of Child-bearing Age who Smoke[†]

Effect		Logistic Regression Results			
		*Estimate**	*Standard Error*	*Chi-Square*	*Prob*
Intercept		-1.5665	0.1581	98.12	0.0000
Medical-Card Status	Yes	0.2633	0.0945	7.77	0.0053
Urban/Rural	Rural	-0.2453	0.0972	6.36	0.0117
Smoked during previous Pregnancy?	Yes	1.4899	0.1547	92.77	0.0000

† The levels of the dependent variable in this model are "Would/would not smoke during future pregnancy". "Would smoke" is the first category and therefore the category for which the model predicts probabilities; those for the second category "Would not smoke" are calculated by subtraction.

* The sum of the parameter estimates for a combination of characteristics yields the logit of the probability from which the probabilities associated with each level of the response variable can be calculated. Under the modelling process used, the parameter estimates sum to zero for each independent variable. Therefore the estimates for the levels of the independent variables not reported in the table (not having a medical card, living in an urban area and not having smoked during a previous pregnancy) are calculated by subtraction.

Table A3: Analysis of Drinking Intention During a Future Pregnancy for Women of Child-bearing Age who Drink[†]

Effect			Logistic Regression Results			
			Estimate*	Standard Error	Chi-Square	Prob
Intercept		1	-1.6468	0.1453	128.44	0.0000
		2	-0.7391	0.1000	54.63	0.0000
Mother or not	Mother	1	0.3717	0.1219	9.29	0.0023
		2	0.1423	0.0767	3.44	0.0635
Employment Status	Full-time	1	-0.2967	0.1860	2.54	0.1108
		2	0.2095	0.1217	2.96	0.0853
	Part-time	1	0.0217	0.2674	0.01	0.9352
		2	-0.2143	0.2076	1.07	0.3018
	Unemployed	1	-0.1528	0.3170	0.23	0.6297
		2	-0.4910	0.2384	4.24	0.0395
	Home Duties	1	0.2308	0.1935	1.42	0.2330
		2	0.0734	0.1408	0.27	0.6023

† For each effect there are two parameter estimates, one for each of the first two categories of the response variable, i.e. 1. "Would continue drinking as usual" and 2. "Would cut down". These estimates, when combined with the intercept estimates produce the logits of the predicted probabilities for the first two categories from which the predicted probabilities can be calculated. Predicted probabilities for the third category — "Would give up" — are then calculated by subtraction.

* The sum of the parameter estimates for a combination of characteristics yields the logit of the probability from which the probabilities associated with each level of the response variable can be calculated. Under the modelling process used, the parameter estimates sum to zero for each independent variable. Therefore the estimates for the levels of the independent variables not reported in the table (not a mother and the "Other" employment category) are calculated by subtraction.

Table A4: Analysis of the Accessibility of Family Planning Advice[†]

Effect			Logistic Regression Results			
			Estimate*	Standard Error	Chi-Square	Prob
Intercept		1	0.9542	0.1039	84.27	0.0000
		2	0.4396	0.1161	14.34	0.0002
Age Group	18–24	1	0.0376	0.1372	0.07	0.7842
		2	0.0093	0.1540	0.00	0.9517
	25–29	1	0.2906	0.1446	4.04	0.0445
		2	0.5348	0.1531	12.20	0.0005
	30–34	1	0.5493	0.1475	13.88	0.0002
		2	0.5735	0.1579	13.19	0.0003
	35–39	1	0.2087	0.1350	2.39	0.1221
		2	0.0446	0.1497	0.09	0.7656
	40–44	1	0.3649	0.1507	5.86	0.0155
		2	0.3324	0.1618	4.22	0.0399
	45–49	1	-0.2452	0.1458	2.83	0.0926
		2	-0.0304	0.1543	0.04	0.8439
	50–54	1	-0.1703	0.1593	1.14	0.2851
		2	-0.3578	0.1807	3.92	0.0476
Employment Status	Full-time	1	-0.3569	0.1166	9.37	0.0022
		2	-0.3303	0.1299	6.46	0.0110
	Part-time	1	0.4455	0.2063	4.66	0.0308
		2	0.2805	0.2280	1.51	0.2185
	Unemployed	1	-0.2399	0.2135	1.26	0.2612
		2	-0.0511	0.2296	0.05	0.8238
	Home Duties	1	0.2022	0.1200	2.84	0.0920
		2	0.2169	0.1334	2.64	0.1040
Health Board	Eastern	1	-0.1304	0.1137	1.32	0.2514
		2	-0.0705	0.1282	0.30	0.5824
	Midland	1	-0.1223	0.1830	0.45	0.5040
		2	-0.5747	0.2130	7.28	0.0070
	Mid-Western	1	0.3595	0.1821	3.90	0.0484
		2	0.3054	0.1910	2.56	0.1098
	North Eastern	1	-0.7947	0.1567	25.72	0.0000
		2	-0.2704	0.1574	2.95	0.0858
	North Western	1	0.2731	0.1934	1.99	0.1581
		2	-0.2651	0.2139	1.54	0.2152
	Southern	1	0.4750	0.1485	10.23	0.0014
		2	0.4706	0.1581	8.86	0.0029
	South Eastern	1	-0.3402	0.1790	3.61	0.0574
		2	0.3074	0.1818	2.86	0.0909
	Rural	1	-0.1710	0.0685	6.23	0.0126
		2	0.2738	0.0731	14.03	0.0002

†   For each effect there are two parameters estimated, one for each of the first two categories of the response variable, i.e. 1. "Yes" and 2. "No". These estimates, when combined with the intercept estimates produce the logits of the predicted probabilities for the first two categories from which the predicted probabilities can be calculated. Predicted probabilities for the third category, i.e. "Don't know", are then calculated by subtraction.

*   The sum of the parameter estimates for a combination of characteristics yields the logit of the probability from which the probabilities associated with each level of the response variable can be calculated. Under the modelling process used, the parameter estimates sum to zero for each independent variable. Therefore the estimates for the levels of the independent variables not reported in the table (age group 55–60, the "Other'" employment category, living in the Western Health Board and living in an urban area) are calculated by subtraction.

Table A5: Analysis of the Probability of Using Family Planning[†]

Effect		Estimate*	Standard Error	Chi-square	Prob
		Logistic Regression Results			
Age Group	18–24	-1.8667	0.2520	54.85	0.0000
	25–29	-1.2613	0.1606	61.65	0.0000
	30–34	-0.8169	0.1307	39.04	0.0000
	35–39	-0.3338	0.1237	7.28	0.0070
	40–44	0.0728	0.1283	0.32	0.5703
	45–49	0.3722	0.1359	7.50	0.0062
	50–54	1.4077	0.1607	76.78	0.0000
Health Board	Eastern	-0.4288	0.0959	19.98	0.0000
	Midland	0.0928	0.1899	0.24	0.6251
	Mid-Western	-0.1547	0.1717	0.81	0.3675
	North Eastern	0.4876	0.1618	9.08	0.0026
	North Western	0.0739	0.1863	0.16	0.6915
	Southern	-0.2568	0.1403	3.35	0.0673
	South Eastern	-0.1340	0.1716	0.61	0.4348
No. of Children		-0.1957	0.0198	97.91	0.0000

†   The levels of the dependent variable in this model are "Don't use/use Family Planning". "Don't use" is the first category and therefore the category for which the model predicts probabilities; those for the second category "Use Family Planning" are calculated by subtraction.

*   The sum of the parameter estimates for a combination of characteristics yields the logit of the probability from which the probabilities associated with each level of the response variable can be calculated. Under the modelling process used, the parameter estimates sum to zero for each independent variable. Therefore the estimates for the levels of the independent variables not reported in the table (age group 55–60 and residents of the Western Health Board) are calculated by subtraction.

Table A6: Analysis of Uptake of Hormone Replacement Therapy.[†] Have Women Taken HRT?

Effect		Logistic Regression Results			
		*Estimate**	*Standard Error*	*Chi-square*	*Prob*
Intercept		-1.7146	0.1209	201.07	0.0000
Age Group	45–49	-0.2763	0.1343	4.23	0.03936
	50–54	0.4027	0.1308	9.47	0.0021
Health Board	Eastern	0.6840	0.1718	15.84	0.0001
	Midland	-0.0103	0.3653	0.00	0.9774
	Mid-Western	-0.0873	0.3085	0.08	0.7773
	North Eastern	0.0881	0.3031	0.08	0.7713
	North Western	-0.1937	0.3664	0.28	0.5971
	Southern	0.4266	0.2279	3.51	0.0612
	South Eastern	-0.4256	0.3871	1.21	0.2715

† The levels of the dependent variable in this model are "Have/have not taken HRT". "Have taken HRT" is the first category and therefore the category for which the model predicts probabilities; those for the second category "Have not taken HRT" are calculated by subtraction.

* The sum of the parameter estimates for a combination of characteristics yields the logit of the probability from which the probabilities associated with each level of the response variable can be calculated. Under the modelling process used, the parameter estimates sum to zero for each independent variable. Therefore the estimates for the levels of the independent variables not reported in the table (age group 55–60 and residents of the Western Health Board) are calculated by subtraction.

Table A7: Attendance at Antenatal Classes[†]

Effect		Logistic Regression Results			
		Estimate*	Standard Error	Chi-square	Prob
Intercept		- 1.0937	0.0950	132.41	0.0000
Age Group	18–24	0.3666	0.2566	2.04	0.1531
	25–29	0.9291	0.1541	36.35	0.0000
	30–34	0.8342	0.1240	45.23	0.0000
	35–39	0.4067	0.1207	11.36	0.0008
	40–44	- 0.0889	0.1314	0.46	0.4985
	45–49	- 0.5485	0.1555	12.45	0.0004
	50–54	- 0.6981	0.1856	14.15	0.0002
Medical-Card Status	Yes	- 0.3637	0.0652	31.13	0.0000
Education Level	Primary	- 0.6635	0.1272	27.22	0.0000
	Inter Cert.	- 0.2614	0.1094	5.71	0.0169
	Leaving Cert.	0.0384	0.1060	0.13	0.7169
	RTC	0.2606	0.2261	1.33	0.2491
Health Board	Eastern	0.6686	0.1008	44.03	0.0000
	Midland	- 0.4103	0.2150	3.64	0.0564
	Mid-Western	- 0.1725	0.1832	0.89	0.3463
	North Eastern	-0.2385	0.1849	1.66	0.1972
	North Western	0.4880	0.1856	6.91	0.0086
	Southern	- 0.1046	0.1456	0.52	0.4725
	South Eastern	0.0773	0.1765	0.19	0.6614

† The levels of the dependent variable in this model are "Attended/did not attend antenatal classes in preparation for birth of last baby". "Attended" is the first category and therefore the category for which the model predicts probabilities; those for the second category "Did not attend" are calculated by subtraction.

* The sum of the parameter estimates for a combination of characteristics yields the logit of the probability from which the probabilities associated with each level of the response variable can be calculated. Under the modelling process used, the parameter estimates sum to zero for each independent variable. Therefore the estimates for the levels of the independent variables not reported in the table (age group 55–60, not having a medical card, having a university education and residents of the Western Health Board) are calculated by subtraction.

Table A8: Analysis of Breast-feeding Behaviour — Mothers with More than One Child[†]

Effect			Logistic Regression Results			
			Estimate*	Standard Error	Chi-Square	Prob
Intercept		1	-1.7551	0.2503	49.16	0.0000
		2	-1.8766	0.2170	74.81	0.0000
		3	-1.2709	0.2421	27.55	0.0000
Age Group	18–24	1	0.1032	0.6536	0.02	0.8745
		2	0.0886	0.6312	0.02	0.8884
		3	-0.1758	0.7202	0.06	0.8071
	25–29	1	-0.8667	0.4080	4.51	0.0337
		2	-0.1259	0.3122	0.16	0.6869
		3	-0.2215	0.3030	0.53	0.4648
	30–34	1	-0.0855	0.2384	0.13	0.7199
		2	-0.3480	0.2463	2.00	0.1577
		3	0.1039	0.2060	0.25	0.6141
	35–39	1	0.3029	0.2058	2.17	0.1410
		2	0.1729	0.1968	0.77	0.3797
		3	0.3821	0.1867	4.19	0.0407
	40–44	1	0.0660	0.2234	0.09	0.7677
		2	0.3768	0.1851	4.14	0.0418
		3	0.5266	0.1917	7.54	0.0060
	45–49	1	-0.4127	0.2481	2.77	0.0962
		2	0.0155	0.1958	0.01	0.9368
		3	-0.5062	0.2378	4.53	0.0333
	50–54	1	0.2720	0.2430	1.25	0.2631
		2	-0.0709	0.2240	0.00	0.9748
		3	0.1023	0.2460	0.17	0.6775
Antenatal Classes	Yes	1	0.2238	0.1004	4.97	0.0258
		2	0.2485	0.0922	7.27	0.0070
		3	0.5102	0.0824	38.36	0.0000
Education Level	Primary	1	-0.6245	0.2132	8.58	0.0034
		2	-0.4664	0.1803	6.69	0.0097
		3	-1.2063	0.2134	31.94	0.0000
	Inter Cert.	1	0.0601	0.1822	0.11	0.7415
		2	-0.2149	0.1640	1.72	0.1903
		3	-0.4307	0.1652	6.80	0.0091
	Leaving Cert.	1	-0.1098	0.1844	0.35	0.5518
		2	-0.3615	0.1657	4.76	0.0292
		3	0.2375	0.1445	2.70	0.1003
	RTC	1	0.4952	0.4013	1.52	0.2172
		2	0.8071	0.3301	5.98	0.0145
		3	0.6566	0.3269	4.03	0.0446
Social Class	Higher Prof.	1	0.6207	0.2565	5.86	0.0155
		2	0.8872	0.2249	15.56	0.0001
		3	0.8941	0.2086	18.37	0.0000
	Lower Prof.	1	0.0508	0.1891	0.07	0.7882
		2	0.2280	0.1658	1.89	0.1691
		3	0.4601	0.1583	8.44	0.0037
	Non-Manual	1	0.0167	0.1637	0.01	0.9189
		2	-0.1744	0.1571	1.23	0.2669
		3	-0.0567	0.1553	0.13	0.7152
	Skilled-Manual	1	-0.3246	0.2084	2.42	0.1194
		2	0.0120	0.1658	0.01	0.9425
		3	-0.3519	0.2099	2.81	0.0936
	Semi-Skilled	1	0.0694	0.1942	0.13	0.7209
		2	-0.5661	0.2026	7.81	0.0052
		3	-0.7085	0.2446	8.39	0.0038
No. of Children		1	0.0768	0.0528	2.12	0.1455
		2	0.2190	0.0436	25.25	0.0000
		3	0.0746	0.0552	1.83	0.1763

† For each level of each independent variable there are three parameters estimated, one for each of the first three categories of the response variable, i.e., breast-fed, 1. first baby, 2. some babies, 3. all babies. These estimates when combined with the estimates for all the characteristics produce the logits of the predicted probabilities for the first three categories, from which the predicted probabilities can be calculated. Predicted probabilities for the fourth category, i.e., never breast-fed, are then calculated by subtraction.

* The sum of the parameter estimates for a combination of characteristics yields the logit of the probability from which the probabilities associated with each level of the response variable can be calculated. Under the modelling process used the parameter estimates sum to zero for each independent variable — therefore the estimates for the levels of the independent variables not reported in the table (age group 55–60, not having attended antenatal classes, having a university education and social class unskilled) are calculated by subtraction.

References

Abma, J.C. and Mott, F.L. (1991): "Substance Use and Prenatal Care During Pregnancy Among Young Women", *Family Planning Perspectives*, 23(3) May/June.

Alexy, B. and Carter, Martin, A. (1994): "Breastfeeding: Perceived Barriers and Benefits/Enhancers in a Rural and Urban Setting", *Public Health Nursing*, 11(4).

Bosio, P.M., Clarke, T.A., McCarthy, A. and Darling, M.R.N. (1996): "Survey of Patient Satisfaction with Maternity and Newborn Paediatric Services at an Obstetrical Hospital", *Journal of the Irish Colleges of Physicians and Surgeons*, 25(1), January.

Bergman, A.B. and Wiesner, L.A. (1976): "Relationship of Passive Smoking to Sudden Infant Death Syndrome", *Pediatrics*, 58.

Berman, B. and Gritz, E.R. (1991): "Women and Smoking: Current Trends and Issues for the 1990s", *Journal of Substance Abuse*, 3.

Bolumar, F., Rebagliato, M., Hernandez-Aguado, I. and Du V Flory, C. (1994): "Smoking and Drinking Habits Before and During Pregnancy in Spanish Women", *Journal of Epidemiology and Community Health*, 48.

Bonati, M. and Fellin, G. (1991): "Changes in Smoking and Drinking Behaviour Before and During Pregnancy in Italian Mothers: Implications for Public Health Intervention", *International Journal of Epidemiology*, 20(4).

Brosky, G. (1995): "Why Do Pregnant Women Smoke and Can We Help Them Quit?", *Canadian Medical Association Journal*, January.

Bruce, N.G., Khan, Z. and Olsen, N.D.L. (1991): "Hospital and Other Influences on the Uptake and Maintenance of Breast Feeding: The Development of Infant Feeding Policy in a District", *Public Health*, 105.

Campion, P., Owen, L., McNeill, A. and McGuire, C. (1994): "Evaluation of a Mass Media Campaign on Smoking and Pregnancy" *Addiction*, 89.

Casiro, O.G., Stanwick, R.S., Pelch, A. and the Child Health Committee, Manitoba Medical Association (1994): "Public Awareness of the Risks of Drinking Alcohol During Pregnancy: The Effects of a Television Campaign" *Canadian Journal of Public Health*, January–February,.

Chalmers, B. and McIntyre, J. (1994): "Do Antenatal Classes Have a Place in Modern Obstetric Care?", *J. Psychom. Obstet. Gynaecol.*, 15: 119–123.

Clissold, T.L., Hopkins, W.G. and Seddon, R.J. (1991): "Lifestyle Behaviours During Pregnancy", *New Zealand Medical Journal*, March.

Cnattingius, S., Lindmark, G. and Meirik, O. (1992): "Who Continues to Smoke While Pregnant", *Journal of Epidemiology and Community Health*, 46.

Daly, S.F., Kiely, J., Clarke, T.A. and Matthews, T.G. (1992): "Alcohol and Cigarette Use in a Pregnant Irish Population" *Irish Medical Journal*, 85(4), December.

Department of Health (1994): *A National Breastfeeding Policy for Ireland*, July.

Department of Health (1994b): *Shaping a Healthier Future: A Strategy for Effective Health Care in the 1990s*, Dublin: Stationery Office.

Department of Health (1995a): *Developing a Policy for Women's Health*. A Discussion Document, Dublin: Stationery Office.

Department of Health (1995b): *Family Planning Policy Guidelines for Health Boards*, March.

Department of Health(1995c): *A Health Promotion Strategy... making the healthier choice the easier choice...*, Dublin: Stationery Office.

Dodds, L. (1995): "Prevalence of Smoking among Pregnant Women in Nova Scotia from 1988 to 1992", *Canadian Medical Association Journal*, January.

Fingerhut, L.A., Kleinman, J.C. and Kendrick, J.S. (1990): "Smoking Before, During, and After Pregnancy", *American Journal of Public Health*, 80(5), May.

Fitzpatrick, C.C., Fitzpatrick, P.E. and Darling, M.R.N. (1994): "Factors Associated with the Decision to Breastfeed among Irish Women", *Irish Medical Journal*, 87(5): September–October.

Formon, S.J. (1987): "Reflections on Infant Feeding in the 1970s and 1980s", *American Journal of Clinical Nutrition*, 46.

Frost, F., Lawrence Cawthorn, M., Tollestrup, K., Kenny, F., Schrager, L.S. and Nordlund, D.J. (1994): "Smoking Prevalence During Pregnancy for Women Who Are and Women Who Are Not Medicaid-funded" *American Journal of Preventive Medicine*, 10(2).

Hanna, E.Z., Faden, V.B. and Dufour, M.C. (1994): "The Motivational Correlates of Drinking, Smoking and Illicit Drug Use During Pregnancy", *Journal of Substance Abuse*, 6.

Haug, K., Aaro, L.E. and Fugeli, P. (1994): "Pregnancy — a Golden Opportunity for Promoting the Cessation of Smoking?", *Scandinavian Journal of Primary Health Care*, 12.

Health Objectives for the Nation (1994): "Cigarette Smoking Among Women in Reproductive Age — United States, 1987-1992", *MMWR*, 43(43), November.

Helsing, E. and Kjaernes, U. (1985): " A Silent Revolution — Changes in Maternity Ward Routines with Regard to Infant Feeding in Norway, 1973–1982", *Acta Paed Scand*, 74.

Howell, F. (1994): "Tobacco Advertising and Coverage of Smoking and Health in Women's Magazines", *Irish Medical Journal*, 87(5), September–October.

Irish Heart Foundation(1994): *Happy Heart National Survey*, Dublin: Irish Heart Foundation.

Keogh, G. and Whelan, B.J. (1986): *A Statistical Analysis of the Irish Electoral Register and its Use for Population Estimation and Sample Surveys*, Dublin: The Economic and Social Research Institute, General Research Series Paper No. 130.

King, G., Barry, L. and Carter, D. (1993): "Smoking Prevalence Among Perinatal Women: The Role of Socioeconomic Status, Race, and Ethnicity", *Connecticut Medicine*, 57(11) November.

Klein, R. and Dumble, L.J. (1994): "Disempowering Midlife Women. The Science and Politics of Hormone Replacement Therapy (HRT)", *Women's Studies International Forum*, 17(4).

Kleinman, J.C., Pierre, M.B. Jr., Madans, J.H., Land, G.H. and Schramm, W.F. (1988): "The Effects of Maternal Smoking on Fetal and Infant Mortality", *American Journal of Epidemiology*, 127.

Lazzaroni, F., Bonassi, S., Magnani, M., Calvi, A., Repetto, E., Serra, G., Podesta, F. and Pearce, N. (1993): "Moderate Maternal Drinking and Outcome of Pregnancy", *European Journal of Epidemiology*, 9(6): November.

Liestol, K., Rosenberg, M. and Wallore, L. (1988): "Breastfeeding Practices in Norway, 1860–1984", *J Biosoc Sci*, 20.

Lindqvist, R. and Aberg, H. (1992): "Smoking Habits Before, During and After Pregnancy among Swedish Women and their Partners in Suburban Stockholm", *Scandinavian Journal of Primary Health Care*, 10.

Link, B.G. and Phelan, J. (1995): "Social Conditions as Fundamental Causes of Death", *Journal of Health and Social Behaviour*, (Extra Issue): 80–94.

Martin, J. and Monk, J. (1980): *Infant Feeding*, London: HMSO.

Matteson, P.S. and Hawkins, J.W. (1993): "What Family Planning Methods Women Use and Why Change Them" *Health Care for Women International*, 14(6).

McSweeney, M. and Kevany, J. (1982): *Infant Feeding Practices in Ireland*, Dublin: Health Education Bureau.

Meredith, H.V. (1975): "Relationship between Tobacco Smoking of Pregnant Women and Body Size of their Progeny: A Compilation and Synthesis of Published Studies", *Human Biology*, 47.

Meyer, L.C., Peacock, J.L., Bland, J.M. and Anderson, H.R. (1994): "Symptoms and Health Problems in Pregnancy: Their Association with Social Factors, Smoking, Alcohol, Caffeine and Attitude to Pregnancy" *Pediatric and Perinatal Epidemiology*, 8.

Michalsen, K.F., Larsen, P.S., Thomsen, B.L. and Samuelson, G. (1994): "The Copenhagen Cohort Study on Infant Nutrition and Growth: Duration of Breast Feeding and Influencing Factors", *Acta Paediatr*, 83.

Midland Health Board (1996): *Report on Family Planning Study conducted on behalf of the Midland Health Board by Lansdowne Market Research Co.*, Tullamore: Midland Health Board.

Milham, S. and Davis, R.L. (1991): "Cigarette Smoking During Pregnancy and Mother's Occupation", *Journal of Occupational Medicine*, 33(4).

Mitchie, S., Marteau, T.M. and Kidd, J. (1990): "Cognitive Predictors of Attendance at Antenatal Classes", *British Journal of Clinical Psychology*, 29: 193–99.

Novotny, R., Kieffer, E.C., Mor, J., Thiele, M. and Nikaido, M. (1994): "Health of Infant is Main Reason for Breast-feeding in a WIC Population in Hawaii", *Journal of the American Dietetic Association*, 94(3), March.

O'Hare, A., Whelan, C.T. and Commins, P. (1991): "The Development of an Irish Census-Based Social Class Scale", *The Economic and Social Review*, 22(2).

Parazzini, F., Dindelli, M., La Vecchia, C. and Liati, P. (1991): "Smoking in Pregnancy: A Survey from Northern Italy", *Soz Praventivmed*, 36.

Pritchard, C.W. (1994): "Depression and Smoking in Pregnancy in Scotland" *Journal of Epidemiology and Community Health*, 48.

Quarles, A., Williams, P.D., Hoyle, D.A., Brimeyer, M. and Williams, A.R. (1994):"Mothers' Intention, Age, Education and the Duration and Management of Breastfeeding", *Maternal-Child Nursing Journal*, 22(3), July–September.